M000289532

Praise for *Last Comforts: Notes From the Forefront of Late Life Care*

"A deeply insightful book that addresses the complex issue of helping individuals who need end-of-life care. Last Comforts presents real life situations and, most importantly, offers solutions, support, and resources."

Steve Saling, resident,
Leonard Florence Center for Living, Chelsea, Massachusetts

"Journalist Ellen Rand embedded herself in the front lines of end-of-life care and became a participant in the quest to transform dying.

"To anyone perplexed by why so many Americans die badly when so many enlightened alternatives exist, Last Comforts provides answers and points the way to tangible solutions.

"Rand's investigative skills and word craft result in a must-read book, not only for healthcare and policy wonks, but more importantly, for any adult child bearing the weight of parent care. Authoritative and highly readable, Last Comforts is at once sobering and hopeful.

"This book should be on the desk of every health care and human service executive, every medical educator, and every legislator across this country."

Ira Byock, MD, Founder and Chief Medical Officer.
Providence Institute for Human Caring;
author of *Dying Well* and *The Best Care Possible*

"Determining what has given meaning to one's life is often a topic of reflection by those approaching the end of their lives. Ellen Rand's personal experiences illustrate how serving others receiving late life care can teach all of us how to live more fully. In this book, baby boomers get to preview what is ahead in their journey."

Greg Schneider, Founder, Hospice Volunteer Association, and CEO, Hospice Educators Affirming Life (HEAL)

Last Comforts

Notes from the Forefront
of Late Life Care

Ellen Rand

Cypress Publishing

Library of Congress Control Number 2015920779
Last Comforts: Notes from the Forefront of Late Life Care / by Ellen Rand

ISBN 13: 978-0-9966153-4-1
ISBN-10: 0 9966 153-4-2

Printed in the United States of America
First Edition, March 2016

Cover artist: Jessica Liu, MD

http://lastcomforts.com/

For orders, contact:
Cypress Publishing
lastcomforts@gmail.com

Dedicated to Simon, Kyla, Sarah, Nicholas, and Carter. The family continues....

Contents

Part Two

Part Three

Foreword

by Stephen C Schimpff, MD

A must read for caregivers, individuals with serious illnesses, their loved ones who care about their care and elected officials. Using the reporter's skill of interviewing, analyzing and explaining, Ellen Rand tells us what does not work today on our path to death and how the "system" can be changed so that we can die with dignity, in comfort and with those we love around us.

She explains why it is time to "tear down the wall" that separates hospice care from palliative care, the wall that separates those who want to continue treating their illness yet would like to die a natural death and the wall that reimburses for all sorts of medical procedures and tests but not for compassionate discussion.

Healing does not need to equate with cure of disease but rather of a spiritual experience despite the ultimate ending of life. To be a healer requires training just as training is required to do an exam, place a catheter or write a prescription. Physicians are all too often untrained and thus unaware of how to be healers despite their desire and intention to be so. Nurses are better equipped by their training but often are too pulled by bureaucratic requirements to have the time needed to be effective. Still, nurses are at the "heart of caring" and their efforts are the ones that most often transform end of life care to a healing experience.

Rand explains why the nursing assistant in a nursing home, ostensibly at the bottom of the professional totem pole, is the key to good compassionate care and why she needs to have the autonomy to be effective. She explains why there is just too much paperwork necessary in hospice care just as there is in all of health care—taking the caregiver's time away from the patient. She describes the lack of training of physicians to engage in meaningful listening conversation about medical care in general and end of life care in particular. And the importance of training in palliative care, empathy, interprofessional collaboration and care coordination.

Rand refers to the studies of physicians who consistently state—contrary to how most physicians actually practice—that they would not want aggressive end of life care but rather a care system more akin to that found in hospice and with good palliative care beforehand.

Importantly, the author understands that for change to occur, it will take the concerted efforts of many, working together. She uses examples of leading politicians who understand what needs to happen but can only make it happen if there is a groundswell of public outcry for change. I am reminded of a phrase from Abraham Lincoln "Public sentiment is everything. With public sentiment, nothing can fail. Without it, nothing can succeed."

—Stephen C Schimpff, MD, internist, professor, former CEO of the University of Maryland Medical Center, and author of *Fixing the Primary Care Crisis: Reclaiming Relationship Medicine and Returning Healthcare Decisions To You And Your Doctor.*

Introduction

" People are less satisfied with care than they were in 2000, and I think it's now urgent for us to start thinking about what interventions we can do to improve care at the end of life given that we are facing a 'silver tsunami.' " —Joan Teno, professor, Brown University School of Public Health in the Journal of Palliative Medicine.[1]

As a hospice volunteer, I once asked a woman I'd been visiting for several months what she wanted for her upcoming 75th birthday. She was a ward of the state and living in a nursing home. Wheelchair-bound, she was in the last stages of metastatic breast cancer. She thought briefly and winked at me.

"Life," she said.

Life. Of course. We all want to live as well as we can for as long as we can. Eventually though, our bodies begin to betray us and we have to reconsider and accept who and how we are in light of these affronts. Many of us aging baby boomers, who have already lost our parents, realize that loss is not confined to the Greatest Generation; it's happening to us. We shudder when hearing bad news about our friends and contemporaries.

Who wants to think about the prospect of the end of life? Who wants to talk about it? Few of us, it seems. But we must. On a personal and societal level, there's no better way to address serious illness, decline, and death.

How will we be cared for in the closing chapters of our lives? There is still time for us, as a society, to figure that out, if we can get over the hurdle of addressing one of the last societal taboos.

The current state of end-of-life care is fragmented, dysfunctional, costly, and unsustainable. That's been exhaustively documented.[2] Too much aggressive care is given that is futile, costly, and ruinous of the quality of the end of people's lives. There's too little talking between physicians and their patients, or between patients and caregivers, on the subject of what truly matters as time grows shorter.

Ironically, all of the medical, technological, and even nutritional advances that have enabled us to live healthier and longer lives have also led to more of us dying older, sicker and with multiple chronic conditions—including dementia—than we would have without the advances. We become less able to care for ourselves as we decline.

As the baby boomer generation lurches—sometimes kicking and screaming—into old age, ten thousand of us become eligible for Medicare each day. By 2030, one-fifth of the population will be 65 and older, compared to 13 percent in 2015. The fastest-growing part of the elderly population is the "oldest old," that is, those who are 85 and above. The "oldest old" will number nine million by 2030, more than twice the size of that population in 2015. Americans requiring long-term care is expected to more than double from 13 million in 2000 to 27 million in 2050.

Last Comforts

This book chronicles my own journey through this unwelcome territory, beginning with the illnesses and loss of my parents and continuing through more than five years as a hospice volunteer. Though I had initially aimed to write solely about hospice, it soon became clear that there were so many broader, interwoven issues in end-of-life care. I broadened my reporting to cover such issues as medical and nursing education, dementia care, long-term care alternatives, challenges faced by minority, gay, and transgender populations, and public policy.

The book grew out of one basic question that kept nagging at me not long after I became a hospice volunteer: Why do people enter into hospice care so late in the course of their illness? So late that they don't have the chance take full advantage of all that hospice offers. So late that there isn't sufficient time to develop the trust, ease and, yes, friendship that can provide great comfort for the ill and their families experiencing what is likely the biggest challenge of their lives. Call it curiosity, call it frustration, call it exercising a reporter's muscles, this question drove me to begin researching the current realities of end-of-life care. I wanted to learn: how can we do this better?

I am an optimist by nature. My goal is to look to the pathfinders and innovations in caring for people with advanced and life-limiting illness to learn how the future might be dramatically different for the coming wave of aging baby boomers.

The seeds for better end-of-life care have been planted. It is up to us to nurture the seeds and insist on the kinds of

Introduction

changes we'll need. On a personal level, we want to make sure that those closest to us understand what we want, particularly if we reach a point when we cannot speak for ourselves.

This is not a definitive history of the hospice and palliative care movements, nor is it an encyclopedia of all of the positive steps already taken. Rather it is a mosaic of the lessons I've learned not only from remarkable professionals who have been my guides along this journey, but also from the people whose lives I've been privileged to be a part of, over the years, and whose names and identifying details have been changed to protect their privacy.

In Part 1, you'll read about people I've met as a volunteer. Their stories illustrate issues central to end-of-life care. Part 2 focuses on innovations and solutions. Part 3 provides practical guidance and resources for those facing serious illness, or caring for those who are.

All professions use acronyms and hospice care is no exception. If an acronym is repeated, it is spelled out as it appears, and it is listed alphabetically in the Appendix.

A word about what you will not find in this book. I have not written about children or pediatric illness. I am a volunteer with Holy Name Medical Center in Teaneck, N.J. Our hospice services do not include care for children with terminal illnesses and their families.

Physician-assisted suicide (or, as its advocates prefer, aid-in-dying) is not addressed in this text, though many people think it is a good solution for some people who are of sound mind but can no longer bear the intractable pain and debility of their illness. Some states are considering legislation allowing it, in addition to the five that already do.

People wish for quick ends for any number of reasons, among them, a fear of being a burden for their loved ones, or fear of the ravages of a relentless illness, as was the case of 29-year-old Brittany Maynard—who had an aggressive brain tumor and chose to end her life with the blessing of her husband and mother.

People in their late eighties and nineties have told me they've lived too long, that they're tired and have had enough. None said they would put an end to their lives if they could.

Unfortunately, the public dialogue on this issue has been a cacophony of vitriol on all sides. Some say we're trampling on everyone's individual rights if we don't have the legal right to assisted suicide. Others rail against the slippery slope we'd create with it. It's all too much heat and not enough light. Assisted suicide is a big distraction from the deeper issue at hand, which is that too many people are bedeviled by fragmented and often futile measures that prolong suffering and add nothing to the quality of life.

Becoming a Hospice Volunteer

Ten years after my father's death in a hospital in 2000, and five years after my mother died in 2005 at home in hospice care, I read a small item in the local newspaper announcing that Holy Name Medical Center was looking for people to sign on for hospice volunteer training. I could do this, I thought.

Introduction

I was drawn to hospice care because of its caring and profoundly respectful philosophy. Its practice offers physical and emotional comfort, support, and kindness to the dying, and to their families. Managing pain and other symptoms is central, but that is only a part of what hospice does. Hospice gives families the time and space to laugh, to cry, to remember, and to mourn as well as to absorb what death is. As a hospice volunteer for more than five years, I am proud of the work I do though it doesn't feel like work. I am part of a team that typically includes a nurse case manager, social worker, health aide, and chaplain.

Centuries old, hospice shares the same linguistic root as "hospitality." In the middle ages, religious orders established hospices for travelers, the ill, or dying, and for pilgrims on their way to religious shrines in Europe and the Mediterranean. Modern hospice care dates back to the mid-20th century, when, in 1967, Dame Cicely Saunders established St. Christopher's Hospice in a London suburb. An English nurse, over time, she became a medical social worker, a writer and, finally, a physician.

Saunders had been working with terminally ill people since 1948 and came to the foundational insight that they suffered from "total pain"—physical, emotional, social and spiritual. St. Christopher's grew out of her long frustration with what she saw as inadequate care for the dying, especially the approach in the medical profession that "there's nothing more we can do."

Dame Saunders visited Yale University in 1963 to lecture about specialized care for the dying. At the invitation of Florence Wald, Dean of the Yale School of Nursing, Saunders joined the faculty as a visitor in the spring of 1965. Three years later, Wald took a sabbatical to work at St. Christopher's. In 1974, Wald, two pediatricians, and a chaplain founded what is now Connecticut Hospice in Branford, Connecticut.

The 1960s and 1970s were a time of dramatic social upheaval. The winds of change that fueled the civil rights movement, the sexual revolution, the anti-war, and the women's rights movements did not leave health care untouched. After women questioned the "medicalization" of childbirth, the idea of childbirth without drugs gained traction. At the same time, a small cadre of nurses and physicians questioned contemporary practices in end-of-life care.

Initially the hospice movement was an all-volunteer effort designed mainly to care for cancer patients. The phrase "palliative care" was not yet part of the lexicon. Long before palliative care became medical and nursing specialties, dedicated pioneers cobbled together basic services aimed at reducing the suffering of the ill and providing comfort—including bereavement support—to their families.

Public support for hospice began with passage of the Medicare hospice benefit law, which was signed by Ronald Reagan to go into effect in 1983. Medicare now covers 87.2 percent of the cost of hospice care. Managed care or private insurance picks up 6.2 percent and Medicaid pays for 3.8 percent. In 1989, the hospice benefit was extended to care for terminally ill people in nursing homes. [3]

Introduction

Hospice is a multi-billion dollar industry. With more than 5,800 hospice programs in the 50 states, Washington DC, Puerto Rico, Guam, and the U.S. Virgin Islands, what began as a largely nonprofit movement has changed too. The private sector accounts for most of the growth, with for-profit hospices making up two-thirds of U.S. programs.

Two of the essential elements of the Medicare hospice benefit have come to haunt us. First, it is based on prognosis in that hospice care is available for a limited time—six months if the illness runs its normal course, although people can be recertified for care if they meet certain conditions. Second, it requires that a person give up any curative treatment. The choice is stark: cure or care. Either/or, but not both.

While regulators continuously tweak the hospice benefit, they have not fundamentally changed its broad outlines since its inception. Cancer is no longer the leading cause of death for people in hospice care. While still prominent, there's also heart disease, chronic obstructive pulmonary disease, stroke, diabetes, kidney disease, and Alzheimer's, not to mention the catch-alls of debility and decline and conditions not otherwise specified (NOS). Hospice was not envisioned to address the needs of the frail elderly living with multiple chronic conditions.

The Canadian surgeon Balfour Mount, a student of Dame Saunders, is credited with being the first to use the term 'palliative care.' Not wishing to use the term 'hospice,' he developed hospital-based services in 1975 at the Royal Victoria Hospital in Montreal, offering non-curative therapy to prevent and relieve suffering and to improve patients' quality of life. Services also included home care and bereavement support.

Palliative care, which evolved from the hospice model, has grown dramatically since the millennium. Palliative care is typically provided in hospitals, as a consultation; it is not widely available in community settings on an outpatient basis. Currently more than 1,700 hospitals in the U.S. have palliative care teams, including more than 60 percent of hospitals with 50 beds or more. [4]

The appeal of palliative care and its great benefit is that you don't have to be diagnosed as dying in order to access it. You can receive palliative care at the same time as curative treatment. If your physician doesn't recommend it, you may ask for a palliative care consultation when diagnosed with any serious illness.

❧❧

Many of us witnessed the trauma of the medicalized version of the death of our parents. Afterward, we decided the story of the end of our own lives would be different.

This discussion comes at a critical time for health care, which is at a crossroads. There seems to be no turning back from the imperative to shift from fee-for-service compensation to payment based on performance and quality. The goals of the Centers for Medicare and Medicaid Services (CMS) are to have 85 percent of all Medicare fee-for-service payments tied to quality or value by 2016, and 90 percent by 2018. Palliative and hospice care will play a key role in what is a tectonic shift in health care. These are reasons to be optimistic

Introduction

about the future, in the words of Ira Byock, M.D., palliative
care pioneer and now chief medical officer at the Providence
Institute for Human Caring, part of Providence Health and
Services in southern California.

At the same time, hospice in the U.S. has reached its
mid-life crisis. It is in need of radical transformation, not in
its philosophy or system of care, but in how its services are
paid for. Advocates believe it is time to design end-of-life benefits based on people's needs, not on their prognosis.

I've come to believe that we have come to a "tear
down this wall" moment in end-of-life care. [5]

It is time for the Centers for Medicare and Medicaid
Services to tear down the wall separating palliative care and
hospice care and to end the tyranny of the six-month cutoff
for eligibility.

Tear down the wall that separates people who still
want to continue treating their illnesses from those who can
accept a natural death.

Tear down the wall that reimburses health care providers for conducting tests, procedures and treatments, but offers
no compensation for a compassionate discussion with a patient and the family about their lives, their hopes, their fears,
their joys and their preferences for how they want to live the
last days of life.

Tear down the wall that prevents our society from paying for the kinds of supports that help the frail elderly and the
seriously ill remain as independent as possible for as long as
possible.

As health care consumers, we must become more

knowledgeable—and vocal— about the kind of care we want for ourselves and for our loved ones. Much of the emphasis has been on the importance of advance directives, and rightly so. We have to learn to communicate better with our physicians, just as they must become more adept at communicating with us.

But there's more we can do. We can raise our voices and use our considerable power in the voting booth to advocate for better health care than we now have. The mills of bureaucracy grind slowly, but politicians and regulators respond to clear shifts in public attitudes. Pressing public policy and social justice issues command the attention of the news media as well as local, state, and national leaders. But End-of-Life? Besides being a topic people are still squeamish about discussing, it is not on the top agenda unless the news cycle is interrupted with a scandal or an egregious case. That has to change.

We must also find better ways to care for people who are ill, whether they are in their own homes, in assisted living, or in skilled nursing homes. That requires better training—and a living wage—for the direct-care workers and nurses who do the work of providing care. Right now, nearly half of home health care workers are on some form of public assistance. That has to change too.

This book represents my journey. But it's yours, too.

Introductory Endnotes

1. David Orenstein. Brown University. "Ratings Decline for End-of-Life Care." May 7, 2015. Surveys taken in 2011–13 reveal people are less satisfied with end-of-life care than they were in 2000. www.futurity.org/end-of-life-care-elderly-915862/

2. Among the many sources: Atul Gawande's excellent book, *Being Mortal: Medicine and What Matters in the End.* New York: Metropolitan Books, 2014; and the Institute of Medicine's report on Dying in America: Improving Quality and Honoring Individual Preferences Near the End of Life. Washington, DC: National Academies Press, 2015.

3. Medicare and hospice statistics: NHPCO Facts & Figures: Hospice Care in America, October 2014, www.NHPCO.org

4. Palliative care statistics: www.capc.org and www.getpalliativecare.org

5. In 1987, President Ronald Reagan famously exhorted Mikhail Gorbachev of the Soviet Union to "tear down this wall" separating East and West Germany. While that clarion call may not have been the precipitating factor, the Berlin Wall did fall two years later, along with the East German government.

1

Friday, August 25, 2000

"Such a long, long time," my mother murmured, teary, stroking my father's face, his arms. She was sitting next to him in the one chair in his darkened hospital room. "Such a long, long time."

This was several minutes after she and I had arrived at the small community hospital in Port Jefferson, Long Island, where my father had spent the better part of his last five months. The doctor had called my mother in mid-morning to let her know that my father's kidneys had failed and they had given him morphine to make him comfortable. It was only a matter of time until he died, though the doctor couldn't predict how long it might be.

"I didn't think it would hit me this hard," she said to me on the way to the hospital, after my long drive from my

3

home in New Jersey to theirs on Long Island.

When we reached my father's room, my body responded before my head did: instantly my heart raced and I felt: no, no, no, no, something is very wrong, this is very different. His arms and chest looked puffed up, filled with fluid, no doubt. His breaths came slowly, as though he was gulping for air. His hands were cold and unresponsive when I held them.

"He's been quiet all morning," said a disembodied man's voice, my father's hospital roommate, unseen behind a curtain.

"Herbert? Herbert?" my mother said, repeatedly. "We're here. Ellen's here. Herbert?" His breaths were coming more slowly. He turned his head toward my mother. Was that a hint of a smile on his face? He made a sound that was low and mournful, like a foghorn at night. It was very, very, quiet in the room. And then, a gurgling sound and no more breaths.

"I think he's dead," my mother said, looking at me, her words more of a question than a statement. Before this could sink in, there was this:

"Mr. Kaplow? Herbert Kaplow?" A woman had entered the room carrying an official-looking clipboard. She was from a hospice organization. One of my father's doctors had finally given the hospital's social services department the okay to contact hospice. With my mother's consent, I had argued, to no avail, in favor of hospice care, most recently two weeks earlier.

"I don't think he's with us anymore," I heard myself tell the woman from hospice. She didn't get my meaning, at first.

4

Friday, August 25, 2000

"I'm so sorry," she said. Shortly after she left, a nurse came in to take my father's blood pressure. There was none, of course. She turned off the IV monitor. The second floor nursing coordinator was the closest this hospital had to a patient advocate. She came in offering condolences to my mother and to me. She hugged me. From somewhere deep in my gut, that's when I started to sob.

"Take as much time as you need," she said, leaving.

Before that day, I probably could not have imagined what it might be like to be present for anyone's death. I would have been fearful of it, which is not surprising: we live in a death-denying culture. Despite the abundance of violent, make-believe deaths that drench our movies, TV shows and bestsellers, we are normally far removed from the reality of death. But that moment in that hospital room was both painful and profound, and it washed away my fears.

I hugged my father for the last time.

We don't come into the world knowing how to deal with the logistics of death. My mother and I wondered, what happens next? The nursing coordinator let us sit in her cubicle while a doctor we didn't know examined my father before he was to be transported downstairs to the morgue. Nurses packed up his things and brought us two plastic bags labeled Patient's Belongings, one containing his leg prosthesis, shoe, and all. That's it? We just leave? Yes. Then somehow, we were out of the hospital, into the sunshine and warmth of a brilliant August day.

A Medicalized Death

One of the reasons I became a hospice volunteer 10 years after my father died was that his last five months convinced me there had to be a better way to achieve a good death. My father's experience may have been unique to him— a Type 2 diabetic, with many of the attendant complications, for half of his 84 years—but it was also representative of so much that is wrong with our health care system.

It wasn't a question of incompetence, malpractice, medical error, or fraud (the pillars of litigation). Rather, the system rendered my father—the voracious reader, the tireless conversationalist, the perennial optimist, the retired attorney who had spent much of his career defending doctors—increasingly weak, confused, fearful, and in pain. My family— my mother, my brother, my husband and I—felt trapped on a careening train, powerless to change the course of events, exhausted, stressed and haunted by my father's suffering.

Diabetes is a nasty disease. In my father's case, its ravages had led to a dozen significant operations over the years, including a quintuple heart bypass and a below-knee amputation in 1987. I joked with him that he ought to do a consumer's guide to hospitals on Long Island, since he'd been to so many of them. Though never a physically courageous person, he always marshaled whatever resources he needed to recover and move forward. After the amputation, it always touched me to see how he accepted with grace people's stares, or matter-of-factly answered children's questions when he removed his prosthesis to swim at the pool in the retirement commu-

6

Friday, August 25, 2000

nity where my parents lived.

In 1999, after his head had cleared from the fog of a mini-stroke, I asked him what he was thinking on his way to the hospital and while he was hospitalized. First, he told me, he wanted the driver to go faster so he could get the help he needed sooner. He wanted to live. Second, he was frustrated because he knew the answers to the questions the doctors posed to him but could not express them verbally.

When the gangrene in his remaining foot began to cause tremendous pain in early 2000, my father gladly took the advice of his podiatrist and vascular surgeon. He entered the hospital for a two-part treatment: a leg bypass, to be followed by partial amputation of his foot. My father's long-time internist was not involved as he did not have privileges at this hospital. My father was assigned to an attending physician who did not know him.

Things do not always go according to plan. The leg bypass was successful, but my father developed pneumonia and anemia. This cascade of events led to August 25.

My father was eating less and less. He developed a bedsore, which never healed and caused him more pain than did any of the operations. He was sleeping much of the time and could not sit up, much less get out of bed, without assistance. Medical indices aside, other indications suggested that the trend was not going in the right direction. When my father was no longer flirting with nurses, or able to read a book or newspaper, I knew he was seriously declining.

I asked the attending physician if my father would qualify for hospice care at that point. "I can't say," was his reply. Can't? Won't? Didn't want to be responsible? It didn't matter. The plan was to discharge him to a rehab center for six weeks to "strengthen" him in preparation for another operation.

Whether he was sufficiently strengthened is debatable, but he did return to the hospital by the end of June. Though weakened, he was still mentally sharp enough to take part in talks with his doctors. He chose to have a partial foot amputation rather than more radical surgery. That surgery was successful, but his wounds did not heal.

One of the biggest problems we faced—and this is all too common for so many families navigating the treacherous waters of serious illness—was the poor communication between the doctors and our family. Email? Out of the question. Phone calls? Rarely returned. Compounding this problem, the three key doctors weren't necessarily communicating—or agreeing—with each other. In short, there was no "quarterback" with overall responsibility for my father's care. Nor was there any final arbiter to appeal to, to reach a resolution. Much of our information came from the nurses, or from the nursing coordinator on my father's hospital floor.

In early August, when it became clear that gangrene had returned, my father was informed that an above-the-knee amputation was scheduled for two days later. That night, I called my father and we talked for 20 minutes, the longest conversation he'd been able to have for a long time. We finally spoke about what had been unmentionable until now. Certainly, none of his doctors had broached the subject of end-of-life options either with him or with the family.

Friday, August 25, 2000

"I've lived a long life," my father said, seemingly ready, finally, to shift to a different kind of care. At my urging, my mother, my brother, and I agreed to meet at the hospital the next morning to stop the surgery. It is common for a daughter to take the lead in health care matters of her aging parents. That was certainly true for us, more so than usual because even though my brother lived closer to my parents on Long Island and could have pulled rank as the older sibling, his bout of rheumatic fever at age 13 had given him a lifelong aversion to doctors and hospitals, or an excuse to avoid them.

My brother did not meet us that morning. My father, mother, and I met with a social services director and then the podiatrist. We asked him to cancel the surgery because we wanted to pursue hospice care.

The podiatrist's fury surprised me. He spit out his words, mostly at me. Medicare wouldn't reimburse home care, he said, because he (the doctor) would not state that a goal could be achieved by sending my father home without surgery. He couldn't say my father was terminal. No nursing home would accept my father because of his open wounds. My mother couldn't take care of him alone. (Never mind that they were fortunate enough to have saved enough to be able to afford home care if needed.) The podiatrist also said that surgery was the only way to get him off antibiotics, which would otherwise destroy his kidneys. Nevertheless, he agreed to cancel the surgery.

Afterward, I sat in my car in the parking lot, shaken, and fighting off tears before heading back to New Jersey.

9

Last Comforts

What happened next also reflected the all-too-common reality that when faced with life-threatening illness, families are not necessarily on the same page at the same time. My mother stayed at the hospital and my brother showed up in the afternoon. He couldn't abide the idea of not "saving" my father, after all. They met with the surgeon. My brother and my emotionally pummeled parents agreed to the surgery, scheduled two days later. My father was fearful about surviving yet another operation, but he was hopeful, always hopeful, about eventually walking with two prostheses. With this latest operation, the surgeon's goal for my father was, simply, "Survival," he told my brother.

My father survived the surgery, as I knew he would, but at a huge cost. He was emaciated and asleep most of the time when he wasn't in pain. Antibiotics were not discontinued. When we visited on Saturday morning, a week after surgery, we learned from a nurse that my father was dehydrated, and the attending physician had ordered hydration and insertion of a feeding tube. This was another bolt from the blue.

The desire to nourish others is basic, I think. We always want to feed the people we love. We honor our heritage and celebrate occasions large and small with delicious foods, served in abundance. It pains us when those we love don't eat. In spite of ourselves, we encourage them to try some food, just a little, just to build up a little strength. But the fact is—and I learned this subsequently from hospice workers—when the body starts to shut down, it does not need nourishment and does not suffer from its absence. This is counter-intuitive, perhaps, but true.

Friday, August 25, 2000

After my father fell back to sleep that Saturday morning, I asked my mother to walk with me. I took her arm and we walked slowly from one hospital corridor to another until we found ourselves in one we hadn't seen before, hushed, with dark wood walls. It was as if we'd stepped into the Twilight Zone.

"What do you want to do?" I asked her, about the feeding tube.

"It seems so pointless," she said. She was beyond exhaustion though we didn't know why until a few weeks later. I was as worried about my mother as I sorrowfully tried to absorb the idea of my life without my father in it.

To me, the idea of a feeding tube seemed pointless and cruel, too, postponing death rather than prolonging life. In fact, my father's advance directive—on file with the hospital—specifically forbade feeding tubes. The attending physician didn't know that, or chose to ignore it. Still, this was a grave and difficult decision to make and its magnitude sank in as we slowly made our way back to the nurses' station.

"Do you realize what's going to happen?" the nursing coordinator asked me, evenly, when I requested that they not do anything until we were able to reach the doctor.

"Yes," I said, just as evenly.

"He's going to die."

"Yes," I said.

The doctor finally called my mother on Monday saying that the latest x-ray showed my father's kidneys were failing. There would be no feeding tube. He promised to make my father as comfortable as possible. With my father's

11

blessing, my brother decamped for his annual visit to a New Hampshire wolf preserve. On Tuesday, my cousin, my son, and I drove to Long Island to pick up my mother and visit my father. He was awake and happy to see us.

When we left the hospital that night, we held on to one another. It was like the finale of the old Mary Tyler Moore show when the entire crew shuffles out, hanging on to one another and singing, unexpectedly, "It's a Long Way to Tipperary." It had been a long way to get to this point, too. We might not have thought so then, but we had said "I love you" to my father for the last time.

October 2, 2005

Four weeks to the day after my father died, my 82-year-old mother underwent surgery for lung cancer. Some months later, she told me she would be glad for two good remaining years for herself. She made us promise there would be no more hospitals. She wanted to end her days at home. She was adamant about what she wanted—or more precisely, what she didn't want—at the end of her life. Despite our crash course in death with my father, I still could not imagine the reality that one day she too would die. But, her openness was a blessing for my brother and me.

My mother recovered well enough from lung surgery to continue to live independently in the sunny two-bedroom condo she loved. She maintained an active social life. She had never learned to drive, but got around nicely by taxi service. We looked for signs of grief or depression after my father's death, but the truth was this. Widowhood suited her. I once asked her if she missed my father.

"No," came the emphatic reply. I refrained from saying that I did. Later on, equally emphatically, she insisted on not wanting to be buried next to him. (They rest diagonally opposite each other now.)

In the spring of 2003, I noticed that bills remained unopened on the kitchen countertop. This was a troubling sign for a woman who believed in paying bills promptly all of her life. She spoke of having nightmares. She started dropping things, and had problems with balance.

By summer, she was diagnosed with a brain tumor. It's never a good thing when a doctor calls and says, "I'm afraid I have bad news." The news was this. My mother had a nodule on the lung and a lesion in the brain. His theory was that the lesion was a metastasis from the lung cancer. He gave me the names of specialists in radiation oncology, neurology, and brain surgery. He'd already given them to my mother, and knew about her "no more treatment" mantra, but pleaded with me to Do Something. In his view, doing nothing was simply not an option. He was concerned and sad. He'd known my parents since they moved to Long Island. After this conversation, though, he handed her case off to the specialists and bowed out of my mother's life.

"I'm finished," my mother said when I called her after speaking with her doctor. She was near tears.

"Maybe not," I said, because denial can be useful sometimes. I promised that whatever lay ahead, we would be with her. And then I shifted into Organizing mode—because

Last Comforts

like so many women, that's how I cope—arranging doctor visits and planning a birthday party for her a week later.

Over the next three weeks, my mother agreed to see various doctors and ultimately decided to go ahead with four weeks of 20 whole-brain radiation treatments. She was determined to attend my niece's upcoming wedding in October, and she did. We didn't know how my mother would be after all the radiation, but since she was determined to stay in her own home, it seemed time for live-in help. Remarkably, she didn't object. In a blur, it seemed, I interviewed prospective aides. Who were these people, really? Who knew if any of their references were legitimate? Can you entrust the life of a person you cherish with a stranger?

We found Lana through a home health-care agency of probably dubious legitimacy, the same agency that had provided aides for my aunt many years earlier, after she'd been diagnosed with ALS. Lana was a smart, trim, middle-aged woman from Belarus who spoke English well and whose no-nonsense demeanor we thought might mesh well with my mother. Under the agency's terms, Lana worked seven days a week, with two days off per month. We didn't question whether that was even legal, but went ahead anyway. Time was of the essence.

At that point, my mother was still mostly herself. The aide and my mother had time to get to know each other well, which they did. As time wore on, Lana became indispensable to my mother; walking with her, when she could still walk, reading novels to her, when she could still pay attention, sharing stories about each other's lives. My mother comforted

Lana, too: one time, my mother held Lana as she cried after hearing about her own father's death a half a world away.

Our lives took on a new rhythm: every Saturday my husband and I drove to Long Island to spend the day with my mother. We gave Lana time off while I went to the supermarket and the bank and cooked dinners for that night and the week ahead. I always loved it when the aroma of roast chicken, or soup, brownies or carrot cake filled the house. It gave us the illusion, if not the reality, of life proceeding normally. During the first year of her illness, I stayed overnight when Lana had time off; my brother spent the rest of the weekend. The second year, my husband and I spent the entire weekend, once a month initially, and then twice a month later on.

Dark humor was one way we coped. "I wonder what's going to get me," my mother once mused, "the lung or the brain?" Or mystery guest number three, I replied. Many months later, my son and I, along with my niece and my cousin, placed bets with each other not only on the date my mother would die, but also on how precisely her illness would administer its final blow. As it turned out, we were all wrong; she outlived all of our fears and expectations.

The radiation did what it was supposed to do, which was to shrink the tumor, but her condition was still incurable. She enrolled in hospice in December 2003. When a nurse came by for her first follow-up visit, I noticed that the first thing she did was to sit on the couch next to my mother and hold her hand, asking how she was. I was struck then—and innumerable times after that—with her kindness and warmth.

15

Last Comforts

Just one small gesture can mean so much.

A hospice nurse once told me that decline—or disease progression, a favored expression—does not take place in a straight line. There's a period of decline, a plateau, decline, plateau. Sometimes the decline is precipitous. Sometimes the plateau lasts quite a while. There are good days and bad days. My mother was relatively stable for some time. She was re-certified for hospice a few times. (Once you're in hospice care, if you live longer than six months, you have to be re-certified. If not, you become, in hospice parlance, a "live discharge.")

When decline came, it was both physical and mental and it's difficult to say which was worse. There was a period of Bizarro Mom, when she spoke in a seemingly different voice, accusing me of selling her furniture, wondering where her real family was, complaining about the motorcycle accident that put her in her current state, claiming she was being held against her will. There was Terrified Mom, which broke my heart, because what she was hallucinating may have seemed metaphorical though it was real to her. Lost in a strange subway station, she didn't have her purse. It was dark and she was afraid. Where should she go and who would meet her? There was Angry Mom, railing against the fates, against my father, against God for doing this to her.

She lost words, phrases, thoughts. She declared she had no mind left, but had oases of clarity, as when I asked, in her last year, how she felt. She said, "Languid."

She could walk less and less and then could barely stand, even with help. For a brief period toward the end of 2004, hospice provided a commode that we set up in the liv-

16

ing room near her couch so she wouldn't have to go as far as the bathroom. She was miserable about it, mortified and disgusted.

A new slew of accoutrements joined the lotions, tissues, and Q-tips on the TV tray: surgical gloves, Baby Wipes, Clorox, flushable toilet cleaners and antibacterial hand cleaners. I learned how to do the shuffling dance of helping my mother up, swiveling her to get her in position over the commode, and helping her down, all the while envisioning us both falling back on the couch, me on top of her, or her tipping over as she sat at an awkward angle. It made me feel inadequate to the task, shaky and exhausted.

The transition from couch and commode to hospital bed and diapers was short. "My last bed," she snarled, as the delivery people assembled it in her living room. The bed sat, like the proverbial elephant in the room, for a day before she agreed to use it. After that, her confusion and hallucinations worsened. A hospice nurse advised that the anti-psychotic Haldol would stop the hallucinations and the paranoia that convinced her she was in a "facility" and being held hostage. The trade-off was that she'd be sleeping more. Better for her to be sleeping than anxious and terrified, I thought.

She kept saying she wanted to die, but her stubborn warrior body and spirit knew otherwise. My bedridden mother struggled for nine more months, sleeping more, eating less, bruising herself trying to escape the bed, picking at sheets and blankets (it's called "terminal agitation" and is extremely common, though I didn't know it at the time), talking to whatever spirits or creatures she was seeing in bed with her.

Last Comforts

Sometimes they were babies; other times they were reptiles attacking her. I sat by her bed, holding her hand, my arm resting on the bed rail until it seemed permanently dented from the rail. For hours on end, it was a combination of tedium and stress. Sometimes it was so quiet in the house that the only sound was the hissing of her air mattress.

At night, particularly when we spent weekends with her, my mind whirred like an electric meter: am I doing the right thing? Should I have taken a little more time to try to get her to eat something? When would this be over? Could things possibly get worse? (Yes.) Saddest of all, I was turning into a person who wished that her mother would die.

The human body is not meant to remain in bed without moving for months at a time. There was a cascade of complications: the beginnings of a bed sore, arm swelling, a brief and unhappy episode with a catheter, a racking, loose cough, stomach pain, back pain, leg cramps and more. Her skin, once so clear and beautiful, became rough and dry. We started to give her morphine, in eyedropper form, from the bottle in a kitchen cabinet, waiting for the right time. Hospice had given us a pamphlet on "Last Days" that outlined the signs of end-stage illness. It was the closest thing to a road map that we had, on what to look for and what to expect. We referred to it regularly, as if trying to decode the mystery that was my mother's illness.

Mid-morning Friday in early October, a nurse called me from my mother's house, after she'd had a particularly awful night. The nurse said my mother had taken a turn, that she was actively dying, and had maybe 24 to 48 hours left.

18

Friday, August 25, 2000

It was the call we had been wishing for, and dreading, for so long and now it was upon us. We quickly packed for the weekend, arranged for the cat's care, called our son and my brother, and headed to Long Island.

Was she comatose? I don't know. Did she squeeze my hand slightly when we arrived and I told her we were there and that her much beloved grandson was coming too? Perhaps. I like to think so. Fortunately, at that point, there was nothing unresolved between us—there was little we hadn't talked about, argued about, or laughed about over the years. We always said, "I love you." She always told me how proud she was of me and that I was her rock. She was mine too.

True to form, my mother lingered past the 48-hour forecast. Shortly after my brother went home on Sunday night (and I am convinced she waited for him to leave, to spare him), her breathing changed and we knew this was it. Some ridiculous crime drama played on TV. I shut it off. My husband believes that my mother was trying to say "No," at the end, but I don't, though that wouldn't have been out of character.

We had gotten used to seeing my mother lying motionless in bed. After she died, the sight of her, gone, did not seem odd to me. Nor was it odd to keep touching her face, or kissing the top of her head. It didn't occur to me or my husband or son or Lana to cover her face. Lana and I hugged each other, for the first time in two years. She and I weren't like family, exactly; it felt more like we had forged a bond side-by-side in combat.

The logistics of death, which had been such a mys-

19

Last Comforts

tery to my mother and me when my father died, now seemed straightforward. First, call hospice, so that a nurse could come to pronounce her dead and flush certain drugs down the toilet, as the law required; then a call to the funeral home to advise them to expect a call from hospice. Finally, gather the clothes and shoes I'd selected for her to be buried in. It was hanging at the front of her closet.

When two men arrived from the funeral home, they asked if we wanted to stay in another room while they took care of my mother. No, we all said, though I admit that seeing them unfold the white body bag and tucking my mother into it was a shock. When they zipped up the bag, I wanted to say, "No, don't do that, she'll suffocate." Ridiculous, I know.

Lana and I followed them out the door and watched as they loaded the van. I remained outside, watching the van's taillights as it left the driveway and wound its way through the streets until I couldn't see it anymore. I waved goodbye, a child's wave. That's when I hugged myself and wept.

I think the word "closure" should be banished from our lexicon. There isn't any such thing, as far as I'm concerned. Loss is a permanent reality. I think there is something deeper than "closure." It is called solace, acceptance, a kind of absorbing of loss into your being, a sense of completeness. In time, the joys of life outshine the pain. Pleasures large and small become sweeter. When I think about my mother now, I see her in her prime, not how she was in her final months. I think of her quick smile and the hearty laugh that bubbled up in spite of her bouts of sorrow or anger, her warmth and intelligence and the boundless love and affection she had for all of us.

Hospice gave us the gift of helping us take care of my mother in her own home, where we had the time and space to be family (with all its attendant ups and downs). Hospice gave us the guidance we needed to navigate this unwelcome territory; and it gave us the ability to grieve and heal without anger, guilt, or self-recrimination. Experiencing so viscerally the difference between my father's end and my mother's underscored my decision, five years after my mother died, to become a hospice volunteer myself.

2

Training and Reality

It was a bone-chilling February evening when a small group of would-be volunteers and I gathered in a small, make-shift conference room in what was then the hospice and home care offices of Holy Name Medical Center, the hospital looming across the street. In walked Jan, a tall, middle-aged woman with dark hair. Radiating warmth, she introduced herself as the hospice chaplain and volunteer coordinator.

Hospice services at Holy Name cover Bergen County, [1] a 247-square-mile suburb in the northeast corner of New Jersey, across the Hudson River from New York City. Although the word "affluent" is usually affixed to the name Bergen County, according to the latest census, 7.2 percent of its nearly one-million population live below poverty level (compared to 10.4 percent statewide); 15.8 percent of the population is over age 65 (compared to 14.4 percent statewide). In the course of volunteering, I've visited people in small apartments in public housing complexes, in mansions, and in every type of housing in between, as well as in five of the nursing homes in the county where Holy Name has contracts.

To get acquainted, Jan had us talk about why we wanted to volunteer. Several people wanted to extend their various roles as hospital employees. Then it was my turn. Why, indeed?

The simple answer was this was my way of giving back, after all the help my family had received from hospice when my mother was ill. That was part of it but there was more. I'd been through the struggle, the pain, the confusion, the anger, the sorrow, the precious moments of affection and laughter, the exhaustion of living through my parents' final illnesses—and come through whole to the other side. I felt I could help others navigate through it too.

I am Jewish, though not terribly observant. One of the religion's tenets—*tikkun olam*—repairing the world—has always spoken to me. I thought this could be my small way of repairing the world. I believe that how we live our lives and the good we do in the here and now is what matters. I wanted to feel I could do something useful, something that counted.

As a reporter and writer, I've been able to establish a quick rapport with people I've interviewed, most of the time. My feeling is this. I know my story; I want to hear yours. I know how to listen well and to ask questions. I know how to be comfortable in a quiet moment, not filling the space with chatter but rather, letting people elaborate on a point on their own, in their own conversational rhythm. Plus, I felt that with my professional background, I could help people write their own life stories, as a legacy for their families if they wanted to do that.

What I didn't say during training, not even to myself at the time, was that at 62, my own mortality was beginning to tap me on the shoulder. At that point, my friends and I had begun mourning not just the loss of our parents, but of our contemporaries too. As the famous old Pogo cartoon might have said, now it was us. [2] It was our turn to shudder at the news of grave illness among our friends. How to acknowledge this? How to imagine my own life's end? How to live with meaning and purpose in the face of it?

We didn't talk about that during that first training session, but we did talk about our doubts and fears about volunteering. A radiology technician feared saying something stupid to a family member. He feared not being able to project enough of a positive vibe because, he admitted, at heart he wasn't a positive person. A hospital administrator feared people would reject him because he is Filipino.

I had my own doubts too. Was I really up for this? Would it be too sad and morbid? Hadn't I had enough of dealing with death? Would I, not unlike first-year medical students, begin to imagine that I was suffering every illness I saw? (Wasn't I the same person who read R.D. Laing's The Divided Self in college and thought, "aha! I have ontological insecurity"?) Would people accept me, a Jewish person, or would they insist on seeing someone of their own religion? (As it turned out, that has never been an issue.)

We talked about the role of the volunteer: first and most important, to provide companionship to the ill. Volunteers can also provide a period of respite for the caregiver and may do light household tasks or run an errand for the family, if needed. We do not deal with terminally ill children, a relief to me. We are expected to visit a person at least once a week, for a minimum of two hours. We have to keep track of our hours and submit an activity report once a week because the Centers for Medicare and Medicaid Services (CMS) requires that five percent of total patient-care hours be volunteer activity. No other health service is required to do this to participate in Medicare.

The list of what volunteers cannot and must not do is long, mostly having to do with personal care. We aren't allowed to drive patients anywhere. We aren't allowed to feed people—later on that was amended to include not helping people drink from a glass or straw, either. We're not allowed to move patients, turn them in bed, help them go to the bathroom, or change diapers. We are not permitted to give medication. If people experience sudden pain or another type of crisis, we are to call the caregiver and the nurse case manager.

It seemed an odd kind of role, then. We are neither family nor medical professional nor spiritual counsel. The parameters are so limited that in a dark moment, you might imagine that a volunteer's function is to be a glorified babysitter. Jan quoted the hospice director's notion that volunteers

Training and Reality

are the patient's "last best friend," but that does not seem entirely true to me. After all, don't we just parachute into their homes, or into their nursing home rooms, and after we've spent time chatting, reading to them, playing music (on the smartphone, anyway), holding their hands, or just keeping them company in companionable silence, we're off, leaving it to the caregivers to do the hard work of taking care of their loved ones?

Amid the copious printed material Jan provided for us was an explanation of the signs of the active dying process, so familiar to me from being with my parents. I felt I could recite this sorrowful litany myself: changes in appetite, energy, breathing, urine and bowels, possible agitation and hallucinations and more. [3] It occurred to me, not for the first time, that perhaps the best hospice training I had gotten was my experience with my parents.

Holy Name's training included two three-hour sessions, plus a two-hour general hospital volunteer orientation, in addition to a one-on-one meeting with an experienced hospice volunteer and a field visit with Jan. Before we became "official," there were blood tests—hooray! I am immune to measles, mumps and rubella, having had those diseases as a child—a TB test (which we retake once a year), background checks, checking of references and arranging to get a photo ID.

An experienced volunteer I met with offered eminently practical advice: Always call ahead to reconfirm your visit. Find out if they have dogs. Ask if they want you to answer the phone. Bring a magazine, a bottle of water, and paper towels

Last Comforts

(for drying your hands after you wash them when you arrive at a person's house). She showed me how to fill out a report following a visit. (There's a lot of paperwork involved in hospice, as there seems to be in any health-care enterprise.) We fill in the time of our visit, its length, travel time, and general notes about the visit.

At the orientation meeting, we learned about HIPAA rules. (HIPAA is the acronym for the Health Insurance Portability and Accountability Act that was signed into law in 1996). We also learned about the history of the hospital, the meaning of different codes (there's not just a code blue; there are at least 10 more). At a welcoming lunch following the meeting, I talked with a prospective hospital volunteer, while we waited in line in the cafeteria. She told me she hoped to volunteer in the maternity ward. I told her what I was doing.

"I could never do that," she said, frowning. That was not the first time I'd heard that and it certainly was not the last. That's when I learned, too, that merely mentioning hospice volunteering was almost a guaranteed conversation stopper. You might hear "That's nice," or "I admire you," or "That's really important." Rarely do people want to hear any more about it.

On my field visit, I went out one morning with Jan to see Ceil, age 104. Alert and talkative, Ceil lived upstairs from her son and daughter-in-law in a two-family house. After washing our hands in the kitchen, we said hello to Ceil, who was dressed and sitting at the kitchen table. Except for being hard of hearing, she seemed well that day, sharp and in good spirits and not having any of the breathing problems she often had.

Training and Reality

Jan encouraged her to talk about her upbringing. Ceil was born in Austria, lived, and worked on a farm from the age of six. She came to the U.S. at 17. In her role as chaplain, Jan prayed for Ceil with her hand extended over Ceil's bowed head. She read the 23rd Psalm, which I remembered well from sixth grade when my teacher began our day by reading it, every day, before doing so was disallowed in public schools. We left after exchanging pleasantries with Ceil's son. Jan promised that a priest would visit to offer communion to Ceil before Easter.

Several months from the day I started the training program, it was time for my first solo visit. John was in his nineties and had Parkinson's and dementia but mainly I was to be supportive to his wife Ann. John and Ann lived in a tidy, modest house not far from Teaneck. Mary, a short, slight, and friendly woman, greeted me at the door. There was no vestibule. I entered the living room where John sat in a big reclining chair watching TV. His hospital bed was set up in the dining room.

I said hello to John. Ann invited me to join her on the couch. John dozed off, once or twice saying something to Ann that she couldn't hear and couldn't understand. She told me how he got angry when she didn't understand him, though the hospice nurse had assured her that it's common not to understand what people are saying at this stage. She praised hospice—"They can't do enough for you," she said.

John's aide, Lena, stolid and unsmiling, sat with us in the living room. I was sure she was skeptical about me, why I was there, of what use I might be. (My mother's long-time aide Lana was skeptical too about hospice nurses and hospice aides during my mother's illness.)

Ann offered me water and candy. I laughed and declined, telling her I had a wedding to go to in a couple of weeks and a dress I needed to fit into. She asked about me: Do I live in Teaneck? What do I do as a volunteer? She knew I was a newbie. I babbled on (or at least it felt like I was babbling on) about how long my husband and I have lived here—since 1980, when we moved here from a high-rise apartment in West New York, NJ when our son was not quite two years old. She told me her story. She'd grown up in Jersey City, moved with John to this house in 1956, raised their three kids here and now they have 10 grandchildren.

When I asked if there was anything she'd like to do, she said she had to walk with a cane and had to hold on to someone while walking. She wanted to walk when the weather was nice. I thought I could help her with this during our next visit.

She told me how wonderful Lena was, how she did everything that needed to be done. I told Ann and Lena that my family was lucky to have had Lana take care of my mother for more than two years, and what a godsend that was, how we could not have managed without her. I said how important she was to my mother. (All true.) With that, there seemed to be a very slight thaw coming from Lena's part of the living room.

"Was she Russian?" Lena asked.

"From Belarus," I said.

With some pride, Lena replied that she was Armenian.

Training and Reality

Neither Ann nor Lena needed nor wanted to go out. It turned out to be just a "get acquainted" visit. Not able to do anything for them made me feel awkward and superfluous. When the time seemed right, I got ready to leave. We agreed that I would call the following Monday to set up a regular schedule for visits. Ann said she preferred to take things one step at a time.

I think she was feeling overwhelmed, which seemed entirely understandable. When you first enter a hospice program, which John and Ann had done the week before, there seems like a large cast of characters to meet, and not necessarily all at once: nurse, social worker, home health aide, chaplain and if you choose, a volunteer. There's plenty of paperwork. There are pharmacy deliveries. It was a lot to take in, even if you weren't exhausted and stressed from caring for a mortally ill spouse whom you've loved and with whom you've spent all of your adult life.

I gave Ann my phone number and said I'd call her. Before leaving, I went over to John to tell him how nice it was to meet him. Although he had no clue as to who I was or why I was there, he waved and pleasantly said goodbye.

Next time I spoke with Ann, she declined a visit for that week, worried that John wasn't eating. She didn't want to leave him, not even for a short walk around the block. We scheduled a visit for the week after. She called to cancel. There was fluid in John's lungs. A few days later Jan called to say John had died.

Ideally, you'd want to get to know people over time, to make a real connection. Ideally, even over six months, a pa-

31

tient and family can get the most benefit from what hospice is all about: caring for the whole person; offering comfort, pain management, emotional support to enable you to live the best life possible until the very end. A few days? A few weeks? Not terribly helpful, it seemed to me.

Maybe next time, I thought. My next assignment was to visit with Cora, so her daughter, Cora's caregiver, could keep a doctor's appointment. Cora lived on the second floor of a small garden apartment near Teaneck. The day I visited, she was resting in a hospital bed, semi-sleeping and looking jaundiced, with a morphine patch on her right arm. Cora's daughter had already left for her appointment, but Cora's aide was there. Before the aide left, she told me that Cora had only been sipping ginger ale or a shake, better from a spoon than a straw. And that every 15 minutes or so she wanted her position shifted. She also told me that she found it hard to understand when Cora was talking because it sounded like gibberish

"So what do you do?" I asked. The aide shrugged. "Talk about other things," she said. She shifted Cora's position in bed before leaving.

Cora dozed, with the Food Network on in the background. As Ina Garten prepared what looked like a complicated dessert, I looked around the small living room. Pictures of two young boys and several images of John Wayne hung on the wall along with a print of an archer aiming either for the sky or at either a witchy face or spider web. Just as I was trying to make sense of that print, Cora moaned. I shifted her slightly and offered water. (At that time, we could still offer something to drink.) I think she said she wanted water RIGHT NOW (those two words were certainly clear enough) so I got some water; she grasped the spoon and took a couple of sips. Later as I stood by her side, she mumbled something and all I could make out was "trying so hard." As if she was telling someone she's trying really hard to do something. To stay or to leave?

A little while later, Cora became agitated and removed the top of her sleeveless blouse; I put it back up. It reminded me of the way my mother, in her last months, constantly played with her bed covers, bunching them up, so unsettling to watch. Cora asked for her daughter. Several times, I explained that Emily was at the doctor and would soon return. She reached for my arm to help her shift position, a simple sign of trust that touched me.

After a while, there were footsteps on the stairs although the sound was different from ordinary rhythm. Emily had a large boot on her foot. We introduced ourselves. I said I was sure her mother was relieved that she was home, since she'd been calling for her.

"Oh, she does that all the time, no matter who's here. Even if I'm here she does that," Emily said. She literally got in Cora's face, cradled her head, asked how she was and did she want some broth? Emily went into the kitchen to make broth. My guess was that Cora didn't particularly want broth or any other food, but it's such a primal thing to want to nourish the one you love that it goes against the grain not to do so.

Emily lived in the apartment next door with one of her grown sons and a nine-year-old granddaughter. She'd been taking care of her mother for 25 years, since Cora had a stroke at 60. I told her she could call me if she needed a break. Without a trace of weariness or bitterness or any other possible side effects of being a long-term caregiver, Emily said, "I'm here most of the time. I just run out in the morning when my mother is asleep. I can let the dog out and do some errands." She had a foot operation scheduled for the following month. I said I could help her then.

As I drove home, feeling inadequate, I thought about Emily's life and responsibilities, which she embraced so cheerfully. It was humbling.

Jan called me a few days later to say Cora died over the weekend. So yes, I had witnessed the "terminal agitation" she was experiencing.

As a hospice volunteer, I was now two for two. After two single visits, life ended, a far cry from what I thought volunteering would be like. I felt like I hadn't done anything useful at all.

❧❧

The longest assignment I had in my first year of volunteering was three months. It was rare to see people for more than a few weeks before they died. It was not uncommon to visit someone only once or twice. Nor was it uncommon to be assigned to a family, to arrange a first visit, and then cancel because the patient died in the interim.

I learned that at Villa Marie Claire, Holy Name Medical Center's 20-person freestanding inpatient hospice, patients might stay a week, or even just a few days before dying. A

Training and Reality

fellow volunteer told me about the time when a patient died just as the ambulance was pulling up to the entrance. The six-month prognosis requirement for hospice eligibility, etched in stone since 1982 when President Ronald Reagan signed the Medicare hospice benefit into law, was rarely reached.

Was Holy Name alone in experiencing this? Was it the luck of the draw? Not at all. National statistics reveal the commonality of the short-term experience with hospice care. While more terminally ill people are entering into hospice now than had been the case five, ten or twenty years ago, they come in at a very late stage in the progression of their disease. Three weeks has been the national average. [4] That is too little time for the ill or their caregivers to benefit fully from the care hospice has to offer.

Why is this? There is a toxic combination of reasons. Many physicians view death as failure and a referral to hospice as giving up. My father's doctors certainly did. Doctors are trained to fix things, to heal, and to prolong life. Acknowledging the reality of death seems anathema to many. That translates into late referrals.

At the same time, it is difficult to make an accurate prognosis. It seemed to be the case with my father. "I couldn't say he's terminal," my father's main physician had told me, two weeks before my father died. People are eligible for hospice care if their illness, following its "natural course," (CMS language) will end in death within six months. When the hospice movement began in the United States, it was intended mainly to help people with cancer. With that disease, physicians could predict the illness trajectory with some ac-

35

curacy, or at least better than they might when treating a frail elder with multiple chronic conditions, as is more often the case now.

Patients and their families bear some responsibility too for not making maximum use of hospice care that is available. Many cannot accept the possibility of death and, like many physicians, they think the word "hospice" means giving up, as well as being synonymous with "brink of death." If there is the possibility that one more round of treatment, one more drug regimen, one more surgery or other intervention might prolong a person's life, one glimmer of a "cure" or at least the hope of staying among the living for just a bit longer, it takes a strong-minded person to say, "No. No more." This is true especially when family and friends urge the person to "keep fighting."

Government policy discourages hospice use too. After more than forty years with the hospice benefit, our health care system still makes it impossible to opt for palliative and hospice care concurrently with curative treatment.

As complex as the reasons are [5] behind families' late adoption of hospice care, even more complex issues complicate end of life experiences. Certainly, the popularity of hospice use has increased over the years. In 2013, nearly half (47.3 percent) of Medicare beneficiaries who died had been in hospice care, up from 46.7 percent in 2012. The National Hospice and Palliative Care Organization (NHPCO) notes the significance in that rise. In 1995, for example, only 17 percent of Medicare beneficiaries, who were dying, used hospice services.

The growing use of hospice is a small part of the story,

however. More than a third (34.5 percent) died or were discharged within one week of admission in 2013, while nearly half—48.8 percent—died within two weeks. Only 9.2 percent were in hospice care for 90 to 179 days in 2013. The median length of stay in hospice in 2013 was 18.5 days, a slight decline from the year before. The average length of stay in hospice in 2013 was 72.6 days.

Why is the average a relatively high 72.6 days, when so many people die within a week or two of entering into hospice care? More people (11.5 percent) were in hospice care longer than 180 days than were in hospice for three to six months. (You can remain in hospice past the initial six-month period if your diagnosis has not changed, you are still not electing curative care, and you continue to decline. You have to be re-certified, as my mother had been several times.)

Many of the people in longer-term hospice care had Alzheimer's (the sixth leading cause of death in this country) or other forms of dementia. Others had COPD, debility, and other conditions classified as known as NOS (not otherwise specified.) According to the Medicare Payment Advisory Commission (MedPAC), a nonpartisan legislative branch agency that provides the U.S. Congress with analysis and policy advice on the Medicare program, more than half of hospice spending in 2012 was for patients with stays exceeding 180 days. [6]

For palliative and hospice care advocates, the subject of cost is, if not unmentionable, certainly not top priority. The main benefit of palliative and hospice care, advocates stress, is that it provides a better quality of life and enables people to live out their days in as much comfort as possible, wherever they choose to be (mostly at home). A secondary benefit, they say, is that such care is cost-effective because it cuts down on the number of hospital admissions and readmissions as well as expensive, futile treatments.

Here are a few costs to consider. In 2013, Medicare paid roughly $15 billion for the 1.3 million Medicare beneficiaries who received hospice care from Medicare-certified providers, a very small percentage of the total Medicare benefits payments of $583 billion that year. In contrast, acute hospitalizations—inpatient care—gobbled up more than $140 billion in 2012.

Still, when hospice stays exceed 180 days, or when there is an unusual number of "live discharges" of patients who leave hospice care because they are no longer declining, it raises eyebrows among the regulators who are hyperattuned to the need to control costs and root out possible fraud. Indeed, there have been numerous egregious examples of hospice agencies (among the growing ranks of for-profit hospice companies) signing up non-terminal patients; or keeping patients in hospice care (mostly in nursing homes) longer than six months. [7]

Just because hospice use has increased over the years does not mean that people don't undergo medical treatment in the months, weeks, and days prior to entering hospice care. In an often-cited research study, [8] Dr. Joan M. Teno and six of her colleagues at Brown University published an article on "Change in End of Life Care for Medicare Beneficiaries: Site of Death, Place of Care and Health Care Transitions" in the

Training and Reality

Journal of the American Medical Association. Transitions refers to changes in the place of care: moving to a nursing home for post-acute rehabilitation after a hospital stay, for example.

The team studied Medicare statistics from 2000, 2005, and 2009. They found that between 2000 and 2009, there was a 23 percent increase in the use of intensive care units in the last 30 days of life; a 48 percent increase in transitions in the last 90 days of life; and a 38 percent increase in transitions to hospice in the final three days of life.

In addition to an increase in treatments, 9 trips to the ICU, and transitions from one care setting to another before people enter hospice care, there is more to consider. For example, between 1998 and 2010, one study documented increases in emotionally troubling symptoms, such as pain, confusion, and depression, during the final year of people's lives. The study, published in the Annals of Medicine, tracked these symptoms over 12 years in the final years of people's lives. It found that pain rose by 12 percent to 61 percent between 1998 and 2010; depression rose from 27 percent to 57 percent by 2010. Periodic confusion increased from 31 percent to 45 percent when the period of study ended. [9]

Volunteer training did not include discussion of public policy. That was something I felt compelled to pursue on my own. More pressing, at first, was another question dancing in my head: was I making any difference at all in the lives of the people I spent time with? If not a glorified babysitter or a "last best friend," who was I, to them?

The answer presented itself not long ago, when my husband and I vacationed in Andalusia in Spain. In a quiet moment at the Alcazar (fortress) of the Christian Monarchs in Cordoba, and while trying to absorb the story of hundreds of years of brutal and convulsive regime changes, we came upon a display of a Roman sarcophagus from the third century.

Consisting of three panels, at the center were two doors, slightly open, leading to Hades. On the right panel was a man (presumably from a noble family, maybe a lawyer) with a male guide—a philosopher perhaps, or a spirit? On the left panel was his wife, symbols of her domestic life at her feet. She was with a female guide. The guides were teaching the man and woman how to leave this world and pass on to the afterlife.

It was a picture of calm, solemnity, and gentleness. The panel of the woman and her stalwart guide moved me deeply, for its sense of sadness and inevitability of leaving behind all that the woman held dear in her day-to-day life.

This is what we do in hospice, I thought. Whether it is for a few weeks or for several months, we offer comfort, consolation, and companionship for people going through the difficult and profound passage from this world to whatever may await us next. As volunteers, we do this one person at a time.

Chapter 2 Endnotes

1. Bergen County statistics: quickfacts.census.gov/qfd/states/34000.html

2. www.thisdayinquotes.com/2011/04/we-have-met-enemy-and-he-is-us.html

3. Brain Hospice is an invaluable resource devoted to care for people with brain tumors though much of its timeline is also relevant for other advanced illnesses. www.brainhospice.com/SymptomTimeline.html

4. Hospice use: National Hospice and Palliative Care Organization. Facts & Figures: Hospice Care in America, October 2014. www.nhpco.org/sites/default/files/public/Statistics_Research/2013_Facts_Figures.pdf

5. Medicare statistics: www.CMS.gov

6. www.medpac.gov/-documents-/data-book

7. Two sources of information about hospice fraud and abuse: projects.huffingtonpost.com/hospice-inc (June 2014); and a multi-part series on the "Business of Dying" beginning in December 2013, in the *Washington Post.* www.washingtonpost.com/sf/business/collection/business-of-dying/ www.washingtonpost.com/business/economy/medicare-rules-create-a-booming-business-in-hospice-care-for-people-who-arent-dying/2013/12/26/4ff75bbe-68c9-11

8. Teno, J.M., Gozalo, P.L., J.P. Bynum, et al. "Change in end-of-life care for Medicare beneficiaries: site of death, place of care, and health care transitions in 2000, 2005, and 2009." *JAMA.* 2013; 309(5):470–7.

Chapter 2 Endnotes

Teno Joan M., Vicki A. Freedman, Judith D. Kasper, Pedro Gozalo, and Vincent Mor. "Is Care for the Dying Improving in the United States?" *Journal of Palliative Medicine*. August 2015, 18(8): 662-6. doi:10.1089/jpm.2015.0039.

9. Singer AE, D. Meeker, J.M. Teno, J. Lynn, J.R. Lunney, K.A. Lorenz. "Symptom Trends in the Last Year of Life from 1998 to 2010: A Cohort Study." Ann Intern Med. 2015;162:175-83. doi:10.7326/M13-1609 www.annals.org/article.aspx?doi=10.7326/M13-1609.

The study used data from the Health and Retirement Study, a nationally representative, longitudinal survey of community-dwelling adults, aged 51 or older (hrsonline.isr.umich.edu/). Using an interview design, HRS collects information after each participant's death from a proxy informant (usually a family member) about that individual's end-of-life experience, including whether the person had any of the following eight symptoms for at least a month during the last year of life: pain, depression, periodic confusion, dyspnea (shortness of breath), severe fatigue, incontinence, anorexia, or frequent vomiting.

3

Two Planets
Coming Together

Illness is a family affair. If you're a middle-aged woman—a
daughter, wife, niece, sibling or a friend—chances are you
will be thrust into the role of caregiver for an elder. Many
families hire aides for part-time or around-the-clock care.
However, the majority of caregivers in this country are un-
paid family members, or friends. Like Paula.

Paula became one of tens of millions of family caregivers after her mother, Helen, was diagnosed with cancer. When
Helen came into the hospice program, Paula moved her into
her suburban Bergen County home for her final months.
Hospice provides weekly visits by nurses, or more frequently,
if needed. Hospice also provides at least one weekly visit by a
home health aide. But, the lion's share of caring for Helen fell
to Paula whose life was already busy as wife and mother to
three teens.

Last Comforts

A mountain of statistics track the economic, social, and personal health implications of family caregiving. Here are a few notable points:

A July 2013 survey by the Pew Research Center reported that four in ten adults are now caring for sick or elderly family members. That care might encompass tasks as relatively simple as buying groceries or managing finances, but it can also include help with what's often referred to as Activities of Daily Living (ADL): bathing, dressing, feeding, toileting, and transferring from bed to wheelchair, for example. Pew referenced a 2012 survey by the AARP Public Policy Institute and the United Hospital Fund that found that, in recent years, the role of family caregivers has "dramatically expanded to include performing medical/nursing tasks of the kind and complexity once only provided in hospitals."

A study in November 2009 by the National Alliance for Caregiving and AARP reported that caregivers spent an average of 20 hours per week helping their loved ones; 13 percent spent 40 hours per week or more. Sixty-six percent of caregivers are women.

The National Alliance for Caregiving and Evercare (now known as Optum Palliative and Hospice Care) reported in March 2009, in a Survey of the Economic Downturn and Its Impact on Family Caregiving, found that the value of the services family caregivers provide for free when caring for older adults, is estimated to be $375 billion a year. That is far more than is spent on home care and nursing home services combined.

When I met Helen and Paula, I thought I would be-

Two Planets Coming Together

come a weekly companion and friend to Helen, but I also thought this would give Paula some much-needed time to take a break, take a walk, run errands, go out to lunch with her husband on his days off, or otherwise take some much-needed time for herself. After all, caregiver burnout looms for all who take care of loved ones, particularly for extended periods. If you don't take care of yourself, you can't take care of anyone else, a physician once reminded me while I was managing my mother's care, work deadlines, and other family obligations.

Here was the irony: Paula didn't want to leave. I could understand her reluctance, during my first visit. It is not easy to leave a loved one in the care of a total stranger. I'm sure Paula wanted some reassurance that I was not an axe murderer. I probably would have done the same thing.

Paula and I shook hands firmly after I'd parked my car in her driveway. Probably in her late forties, she was tall and imposing, her long hair drawn up in a ponytail. From the driveway, I followed her directly into the unfinished and ill-lit basement where Helen's hospital bed was set up close to an old couch and recliner. The bed faced a TV, and a washer and dryer on the opposite wall. Last season's coats hung behind her.

"Wake up, Sleeping Beauty," Paula said to her mother, a slight woman in her eighties who was sitting in bed with her eyes closed.

"I'm so bored!" were Helen's first words to me, after we were introduced. "What are you going to do for me?" she asked, looking clear-eyed at me.

Last Comforts

I told her we could hang out, talk, or maybe I could read to her. I noticed she was reading "Memoirs of a Geisha," and asked if she wanted me to read that to her, but she wasn't interested. She did want to go outside—the basement opened onto a patio in the backyard. After Paula helped her into a wheelchair, we sat around a picnic table on a glorious autumn afternoon. When Paula went inside to get juice for her, I asked Helen to tell me something about her life, what she'd done, what she liked.

She shared a few details, mainly telling me how wonderful and sweet her daughter was, and that she'd lived in Manhattan before she came here. She was glad to be here with Paula and her husband and three grandchildren. Mostly she wanted to know about me and I was happy to share the condensed version of my life. We talked a little about books and movies. She told me The Enchanted Cottage was her favorite movie.

Later that day, I looked it up online. This is what the 1945 movie was about: A homely maid (played by Dorothy McGuire) and a scarred ex-GI (played by Robert Young) meet at the cottage where she works and where he was to spend his honeymoon prior to his war-time accident. The two develop a bond and agree to marry, more out of loneliness than love. The romantic spirit of the cottage, however, overtakes them. They soon begin to look beautiful to each other, but to no one else. As they fall in love, their physical transformation is shown to the audience, too.

Paula told me that Helen had been a secretary at the American Embassy in Cambodia and that, after returning

Two Planets Coming Together

home, she became a legal secretary in New York. She liked hearing about anything travel-related.

The next time I visited, Paula stayed with us, chattering mostly about her kids, hovering over Helen to make sure she was comfortable enough, or asking if she was hungry or thirsty, doing laundry and intermittently yelling upstairs to her dog to shut up. It seemed to me that Paula hid her nervousness and worry about her mother behind a torrent of words and high-pitched laughter.

When Paula left to pick up her kids from school, it seemed suddenly quiet in the basement. I asked Helen again to tell me more about her life. Her mood turned thoughtful.

"Do you ever really know that it's right, before you get married?" she asked, at one point, adding that she'd been married for a little over a year, enough time to get pregnant and give birth. "I don't think I loved my husband," she told me. "I think I probably wanted to get married so I could become a mother.

"And I have not loved a man since. I guess some people aren't meant to have love in their lives," she said.

"Maybe not," I replied, not saying that I was thinking about my how other people—my mother being one—may have love but then it kicks them in the rear. Which would be worse? It made sense that a romantic tale like The Enchanted Cottage was Helen's favorite movie.

"I'm sick of being sick," Helen told me a few weeks later. "I guess it'll be this way until I die." Before I had a chance to respond, Paula stopped folding laundry and rushed over. "No, no, you can't give up! You have to keep fighting!" she said.

Last Comforts

What if Helen didn't want to keep "fighting" her cancer? What if she was being remarkably candid because she wanted to talk about her fears, or her anger at her illness? It seemed so unfair, to expect her to buy into the "battle" and to go along with the notion that she could and would get better if only she wouldn't "give up."

Instead of sharing a moment to acknowledge a sorrowful and difficult truth with her mother, Paula used her words like a shield to ward off the reality of her mother's decline. I remembered something I'd learned in volunteer training. You may not always agree with what patients and caregivers are doing or saying; you would handle things differently yourself. What matters though are "their solutions, not your solutions," Jan had said.

I didn't try to change the course of the conversation. How could I begrudge Paula her own coping style, when so much of Helen's care was on her shoulders?

As autumn progressed, so did Helen's decline. She became more easily fatigued, nodded off at times, developed a loose cough and occasionally had to use oxygen. She didn't have the energy or interest to talk about her own life, but she was still clear-eyed and wanted to see pictures of past vacations my husband and I had taken. Paula set up her husband's laptop computer on the portable bed table. I put in the CDs and then off we went: to Sequoia, Yosemite and Death Valley. Another time it was the Canadian Rockies.

Paula asked me to bring more pictures because Helen enjoyed them so much.

"I'm running out of trips," I joked. One time, when I

Two Planets Coming Together

showed pictures of a coastal cruise near Maine, she asked me how Acadia got its name.

"Let's find out," I said, and after a few false starts managed to figure out how to get online on the laptop and found, of course, all sorts of information and photos about the history of Maine and the battles between the French and English and Colonials and Indians. (For the record, according to the National Park Service, Acadia probably stems from a name given to the area by the explorer, Giovanni Verrazano, when he sailed by in 1524. The shoreline reminded him of a part of Greece called Arcadia.)

"Where else would you like to go?" I asked her, when we were done with Maine.

"Cambodia," she said. We found plenty of images from Cambodia. She asked me to find Battambang, spelling it for me, and then boom, there it was.

It was like finding a key and opening a new door. I was thrilled to find another way to connect with Helen. After a while, Paula asked if Helen was tired.

"No!" she said, emphatically. She told me about the nice train ride from the capital to Battambang. She told me about the monks in orange robes in Siem Reap who banged on pans at six in the morning, waiting for their breakfast that townspeople fed them. We found odd pictures of bamboo "carriages" that run on old rail lines. I drove home that day warmed by what felt like a sudden, unexpected state of grace.

The next week, we returned to Cambodia, to Angkor Wat, and to Ta Prohm mostly. I read commentaries about the history and how the the temples were designed in response to

Last Comforts

the movement of stars. But Helen was noticeably more tired and a little more confused than in earlier weeks. She asked if I had taken the pictures I showed from the Internet.

My visit with Helen before Thanksgiving was very different. She'd had a bad night, awake for much of it with congestion and coughing. She was asleep when I arrived. Paula sat at the foot of her bed. I sat on the reclining chair facing her and we talked. Paula was exhausted but still voluble. She was trying to arrange a visit to Helen's apartment in Manhattan to do a walk-through and close it out, which she had been dreading. She and a friend had been able to clean out the apartment months before this—she thought it would be too difficult to tackle that "after."

Maybe it was the exhaustion, but gradually she seemed more at ease and talked more quietly about how difficult that past few months had been.

"I probably spend about 75 percent of my time with my mother," she told me. "I don't sleep through the night. I sometimes come down here and sleep on the couch."

She admitted that she hated the phrase "disease progression." She got angry and resentful every time she told a nurse about her mother's new symptoms and the nurse explained that it was to be expected; it was "disease progression."

I told Paula that she was amazing, which was true. With some sarcasm, she told me the story of a friend whose mother had been ill; the friend took care of the mother only for her last two weeks and pronounced the experience "great."

50

Two Planets Coming Together

Two weeks. Great. Sure, easy to say, we agreed. Paula and I both understood the weirdness and the "you don't get it-ness" of her friend's comment. I told her about how, when an acquaintance told me something similar about flying out to see her father in his last week and how important and meaningful that was, I wanted to smack her.

There was more: Paula told me how much she hated giving her mother morphine. I told her about the first time I gave my mother morphine, misread the dosage, and gave her more than I should have. I thought, God, I've just killed my mother! (I didn't, of course.) We laughed as only caregiving veterans can.

Not long after Thanksgiving, Helen died. I called Paula a week later to offer my condolences and to find out how she was.

"I'm lonely," she said. "Now who can I yell at?"

She was finding it difficult to talk to her mother's friends, and to the insurance company. Her kids were okay, but got upset when they saw she was upset.

"You know, my mother and I were on two different planets," she said. "The only reason it ever would have happened that we lived together was the cancer."

We talked about getting together for lunch or coffee at some point, but we never have.

❧❧

After that, it was no longer surprising to me when daughters and nieces stayed on when I came to visit. Is it that they cannot or don't want to let go, however briefly? Is it a

51

matter of being proprietary, or in control? Are they concerned about their loved one's possibly saying or doing something embarrassing or strange?

In volunteer training, Jan said that you could usually tell right away who had a good support network and who didn't. When I came to know Muriel, it seemed as though I'd happened upon a social occasion in her open and sunny home: in addition to her live-in aide, at least one of her three daughters was always there, and maybe a friend or a cousin.

At 92, Muriel was still a real presence, a little imperious and willful. A widow, she'd taken up painting in her 60s; her paintings hung from the walls throughout the house. During my first visit, I sat beside Muriel's bed to chat, with her daughter Emily and her aide Theresa joining us in the living room. We talked about food; we talked about clothes— Muriel liked my blouse and asked where I shop. When she seemed to flag, it seemed the right time to leave. By the third week, Theresa told me that Muriel had awakened in the middle of the night convinced that someone was at the door; Theresa had to open the door to show there was no one there. Another time she was convinced she heard a baby crying.

Around that time when I visited, her daughter Carla was there. Carla and I sat next to each other, with Muriel in a chair opposite us. At one point Carla talked about ordering pizza for her family's dinner, adding that maybe she'd make a salad. Muriel launched into a long, convoluted explanation of how to make a salad with a vinegar and oil dressing, to which Carla listened patiently. And there were in-jokes, family jokes

Two Planets Coming Together

I couldn't begin to parse.

Carla joked about how Muriel loved her aide Theresa more than she loved her. Muriel didn't take that as a joke.

"Never, ever think that," she said, getting teary. "I love, love, love, love you."

Carla got up to hug her and whispered, "I love you, too."

I sat there thinking, I shouldn't be here, watching a private moment like this. I felt like a voyeur but later, reflecting on this moment of breathtaking intimacy, I knew I'd been privileged to be there with them.

❧❧

The first time I met Zelda, her appearance was a shock. Almost 99, she had a full head of steel-gray hair. Her skin was smooth and she seemed to be sleeping peacefully but you could barely see her body under the blankets. She was so emaciated, she looked to me like the closest a person could be to death without having died. Her 70-something daughter, Lila, was living with Zelda and caring for her in the three-family house that Zelda's father had built some 80 years earlier.

Zelda did not respond when Lila introduced me to her, nor did she ever respond over the next several weeks when I greeted her on arrival or said goodbye to her when I left. Zelda's silence did not deter Lila from keeping up a constant patter of conversation, punctuated every 10 minutes or so with questions: "Are you hungry, Mom? Are you thirsty?

Last Comforts

Would you like some Jell-O? Would you like a drink? Let me get you some water."

Lila sat by her mother's side in the living room, doting over her, straightening the blankets, combing her hair, patiently holding a glass with a straw in hopes that her mother would drink.

I thought about my own mother, how she seemed to be in a state of suspended animation for so long: there, but not there. For Lila, Zelda was still very much there, no matter how unresponsive. Lila still had her mother. In a way, I envied her, even so many years after I'd lost mine. Most days, but only in my head, I still talk to my mother.

It was not surprising when Lila politely declined my offer to stay with Zelda so she could go out. She'd say, "It's too hot out." Or she'd say she's a little tired herself and would rather stay in. Lila talked to me about her own health issues, her sons, her grandchildren, before fluttering back to her mother: "Are you hungry, Mom? Are you thirsty?"

Zelda died shortly before her 99th birthday. I called Lila to express my condolences and reached voicemail. About a week later, she called me back to thank me.

"You made me feel less alone," she said. She didn't have to tell me how palpable the absence of her mother was going to be.

4

Connecting on a Different Plane

"Only connect," the novelist E. M. Forster wrote in the book *Howards End*.

Connecting is the heart and soul of what we do in hospice; it starts with listening, which guides the content, rhythm, and tenor of our conversations. We connect to the whole person; he or she is not a diagnosis and a cluster of symptoms. Not that conversation needs to be deep and serious, mind you, though that can come, too, over time. If asked, I'm glad to share the mundane details of everyday life: what I'm planning to cook for dinner, how I spent the weekend, how a favorite sports team is doing.

Last Comforts

But how do you connect with people who cannot communicate conventionally? What replaces the connective tissue that is ordinary conversation?

By the time I'd been volunteering for several months, my goal of helping people set down their life stories seemed increasingly unrealistic. Here's what was becoming obvious to me. Besides coming to hospice care very late in the course of their illness, by the time they do, people may be too ill, distracted, uninterested, or suffering dementia on top of physical illness, to be able to have a conventional conversation, much less think about expressing their thoughts and feelings about the arc and meaning of their lives.

I began learning how to communicate differently. Flo, Jack, and Alice were among my notable teachers.

Flo

I met 89-year-old Flo at a new nursing home sprawled across several wooded acres in northern Bergen County. The narrow slate walkway leading from the parking lot to the building entrance seemed like a kind of magical path transporting me from one reality to another.

Flo was in bed. I could see she was once an attractive woman, her light brown hair upswept off her long neck. She was stately looking, even with one bad eye and the right side of her face and neck black and blue, probably the result of two recent falls she'd had, as her niece and caregiver Carol explained. Offering a luminous smile and asking pleasantly about my children, Flo likely thought I was someone she knew.

She spoke so softly it was hard to hear her. Then, she

Connecting on a Different Plane

was off in a conversation with someone unseen, facing the wall next to her bed. She fiddled with the blanket. She kept moving her legs to get them out from under the blanket. She was never still. Carol stayed in a corner of the room, while at one point I read the day's headlines to Flo, making occasional lame jokes that elicited chuckles from Carol.

While Flo dozed for a while, Carol explained that while Flo had family in Nevada, she had no children, and no one had come back east to help out. When Carol was young, Flo had helped care for Carol's mother when she was ill. Carol was now returning the favor. She spent the better part of nearly every day at the nursing home. She reeled off a sad litany of events that had led Flo here: metastatic cancer; delirium following a new regimen of drugs which, when discontinued at Carol's insistence, returned Flo to lucidity for a while; the falls; the swallowing problems. Carol had become the self-appointed sentry, guarding against any further mishaps now that Flo was here.

When she awoke, Flo began gesturing, talking to her unseen guests on the wall. At one point she became alarmed because she thought she'd left something on the stove. She mentioned there was something "poisonous" there.

"I'll take care of it," Carol told her, calmly. "I'll turn it off and I'll get rid of what's there." That reassured Flo.

Time spent visiting in a hospital or a nursing home is an odd thing. It is a suspended reality. An hour can feel like three. And yet, it came as a surprise to me that when the time seemed right to leave, I'd been there for more than two hours. I hugged Carol and told her I'd visit again the following week.

Last Comforts

I took Flo's hand and told her the same thing. She thanked me for coming, thinking, I'm sure, that I was someone else.

When I visited Flo the following week, I had to stay outside her room at first because an aide was attending to her: changing her clothes, brushing her teeth, and transferring her to a large wheelchair. (The chair was fitted with an alarm that sounded every time Flo tried to get out of it. It sounded if she sat forward, too. It was loud and insistent, like a truck alarm when the truck is backing up. It beeped many times in the course of my visit.)

I introduced myself to the nurse who was readying Flo's drugs for the morning. Brisk and outgoing, she asked me about the morning's weather and said she hoped it would be nice on her day off two days later. She asked if I was from hospice. Yes, I replied.

"I believe in hospice," she whispered to me, as though the very word was taboo here. "After seeing what I see here, I've told my kids what I want. Or what I don't want," she said.

Because Flo was more alert that day, the aide wheeled her to the far end of a common room where about a dozen people were already in the middle of a wheelchair exercise period. I pulled up a chair to sit next to her. Flo did none of the ankle circles, raising and lowering of legs, or any of the other exercises, although she lifted her arm and seemed to count along with the physical therapist, as if trying to keep up.

We established that Flo was a Yankees fan, so I told her about an upcoming pitching duel between the Yankees' and Toronto Blue Jays' aces. I told her my husband and I were

Connecting on a Different Plane

going to visit the new Yankee Stadium for the first time that summer when his brother and sister-in-law came to visit from Ohio. I told her about the joy of swimming laps at our local swim club. With an oldies radio station playing in the background, I told her about how, when I was younger, I could tell what song was playing after just a couple of notes. I told her I used to play the piano. As a rule, I am not overly chatty. I am often content with companionable silence. So, this was something of an effort.

In between these tidbits, as in an ordinary conversation, she told me things too, in a soft voice but with great animation and that luminous smile. I couldn't tell you what she was talking about; I couldn't understand a word. At first, I thought I was failing her in a fundamental way.

Our conversations during the month I visited her reminded me of how, when my son was a baby, I'd talk to him and he'd babble back, animated. Clearly, he knew what he was trying to say, but of course I didn't. But I nodded and asked questions and smiled and mirrored his cadences and his mood. Making a connection, it was joyful and fun. With Flo, this was the pattern: I would start on a topic and then she'd be off on a conversation back, with more eye contact as we went on. Uh-huh, yes, I said from time to time, to encourage her. We smiled at each other. She seemed relaxed and cheerful. Were we connecting? I'll never know, but I like to think so.

The last time I saw Flo, when Carol arrived to stay with her aunt for the rest of the day, I summed up what we'd been talking about (or my part of it, anyway). She told me that when Flo was young, she used to swim across the Hudson River and that she too played the piano. I would have liked to have asked Flo about that. But I was beginning to understand that we have to meet people where they are, physically, mentally, emotionally, and not where we'd like them to be or where we imagine they may have been, once.

Jack

Jack took my hand and kissed it. "Hi, Honey," he said. He had no idea who I was, I'm sure, but he brightened whenever I visited him, as I did once a week one winter. This particular nursing home looked shopworn around the edges but it was clean. Televisions blared from most of the rooms I passed as I searched for his room.

This was a typical visit: I would pull up a chair next to Jack, where he was seated in a large rolling chair that reclined. It was a Rolls Royce of a chair—and we held hands.

"Cold," he'd say.

"It's winter. They'll warm up," I'd reply. I would practically have to shout this, close to his right ear, because Jack, in his 90s, was hard of hearing. He also had dementia. And, a catheter. And, compression boots on his feet. The hospice Plan of Care form listed "debility" as the diagnosis.

When I visited him, we talked (mostly I talked) about the day, about how the football Giants were doing. My hand rested on his chest. Invariably he would begin to move it lower. He asked me if I was married. He asked me how old I was. He asked me if I liked to be held. He asked me if my hand on his tummy felt good.

Connecting on a Different Plane

"Do you want to do it?" he'd ask.

"Nah, not today" I would reply.

"I like to talk with you. I like to walk with you," he said. "You're my favorite. I think I'm in love with you."

It made me laugh. "Wow, that was pretty fast," I said, but he didn't get it. Then he'd doze off for a while.

Did he think we'd had sex? Did he think we'd taken romantic walks in the park? Did he think that when my hand was on his tummy that it was some place else?

Dementia, drugs, or maybe both, left Jack in a nether world and although I had no idea where that might have been, it didn't seem altogether unpleasant. Clearly, we had an odd sort of communication, a surreal connection. Maybe it was a comfort to him, to awaken after a short nap, seeing someone smiling at him and holding his hand.

The hospice-nurse case manager had advised me that if he became sexually aggressive, I had permission to tell him, directly, how inappropriate that was and to threaten to leave if he didn't stop. As she, in fact, had told him herself.

But I was never offended. It made me think: illness and drugs have removed Jack's filters and constricted his life in so many ways. What was left was this primal instinct, this drive, this life force. "I'm still alive," it said.

Some people, maybe most, I don't know, might have gotten indignant. Certainly if a peer of mine said half of what Jack said to me in the course of visiting him over a couple of months, I would have responded very differently. But instead, I was fond of Jack and I found it oddly moving.

I tried to ask about his life, his family, what he did

Last Comforts

for a living before he retired. There was a picture of his large family on the dresser, with him and his wife in the center, both in wheelchairs, but I never met them. He told me he used to run a movie theater in upper Manhattan. I could have told him about how I was born not far from there, or about movies I'd seen, or about the film festival I had co-founded, but I knew it wouldn't register.

Once, when I got to his room, an aide was feeding him his pureed lunch, encouraging him to eat. "That's a good boy," she said after each bite. That winter I'd heard other aides at other times talking similarly to their charges: Good girl, you can do it. Good boy, try another bite. As if they were children.

In the background, there was always television. The Price is Right at 11:30, followed by news at noon. The game show is a frenzied affair, a love letter to consumerism, an endless parade of products and travel prizes. Having seen it repeatedly, I realized that I'll never understand how it works. I've also discovered that during the day, the ads are aimed at the very old: motorized scooters, reverse mortgages, life insurance, and Medigap insurance.

The last time I visited Jack, his decline was clear: his barrel chest diminished, his face drawn, his breathing labored. I asked a nurse to put in his oxygen tube, which had slipped out of his nostrils.

"He just takes it out," she said.

He called out, weakly, for "Nurse," while I was there. Did he think I was the nurse? I leaned in close to his ear: "I'm right here," I told him, stroking his brush-cut hair. Every once in a while, he let out a sound that was part moan, part sigh. An aide brought lunch, which I knew he wouldn't eat. He died the next day.

Alice

The first time I met Alice in her nursing home and introduced myself as a volunteer, she croaked, "If you're a volunteer you better feed me!" I would if I could, I told her, and my answer seemed to annoy her. Perhaps not the best start. In her mid-90s, Alice was bedridden. She'd been here for 10 years. Her bed was on the window side of the room but the blinds were always drawn because light hurt her eyes. She was so thin you could barely see the outlines of her body under her blankets. There was barely enough space for a chair next to the bed, mismatched dressers opposite it, an old TV (usually turned off) sitting on top of one of them. Her roommate slept in bed, clutching a stuffed toy raccoon.

Sometimes Alice slept deeply while I kept her company. A "calming presence" is what the hospice activity report, which must be filled out after every visit, calls it. She slept even while a woman in a nearby room shrieked, "Get me out of here!" every couple of minutes.

Once I met Alice's niece Barbara, red-cheeked and friendly, who filled in a few blanks about Alice. She explained that Alice wasn't especially interested in music, or TV or anything. One time when she was visiting, she turned the TV on.

"Am I boring you?" Alice asked.

After Barbara and I had been chatting for a while,

she left to visit a patient in an adjacent room. Agitated, Alice drummed her fingers on her bed tray, and asked, "Where's your friend? I don't see her." It dawned on me that she was talking about Barbara.

"She just stepped out but she'll be back in a little bit," I said.

"I don't like to see friends separated," she said, haltingly, and I could see that it was an effort to talk this much. "It makes me think you'll leave too. I don't want to be alone."

Just like that, so clear, so different from the times when she was confused and mumbling. That hit me like a blow to the solar plexus, because it summed up what's wrong with this place: the many hours people spend alone, fearful and helpless, even when the necessities are taken care of.

"You're not alone," I said. "We're here."

When her niece returned, Alice relaxed.

As time went by, I wondered whether my presence and efforts made any difference to Alice. Was I making her day better, even a little? I couldn't tell.

A few weeks later, before I got to Alice's room, a woman in her wheelchair, in her accustomed place in the hallway opposite Alice's room, told me that Alice had been calling out all day.

"Maybe you can do something," she said.

I barely had time to put down my coat and bag when Alice started talking, in her halting way, but clearly in a panic.

"I'm so sorry that we're alone here and trapped," she said. "It's a dark cave and we're trapped. If we try to leave,

Connecting on a Different Plane

they can chop your head off." She believed I was a family member. She had noticed that her roommate had half-shut the door to the room, when she had gotten up to go to the bathroom. Alice's hands shook.

"Open the door! Open the door!"

I did so, and she told me she was claustrophobic. "Wanda!" she cried out. "Margaret!" Her gaze was locked somewhere over the television set on the dresser. She'd seen "people" in her room before. I thought she might have been seeing the two women she was calling out to.

Her dark eyes fixed on mine, silently imploring. I knew that, to have any hope of providing comfort to Alice, I had to acknowledge her reality but also try to reassure her that she was not in danger.

"We're safe and comfortable and well taken care of," I told Alice, trying to sound calm as she clutched my hands tightly, looking up at me. "We're okay right here."

Although she continued to warn against trying to escape the cave, she gradually calmed down. After a pause, she asked, "Are you the little boy who visited here a few days ago and said you'd be back?"

"I was here last week," I told her. "I played music for you on my phone."

She gave no sign of hearing this.

"Are your parents here?"

"No, they're not."

"We'll wait until your parents get here to pick us up and take us home," she said. So often, when people are close to the end of their lives, they talk about needing to take a trip. Needing to leave. Needing to go home. I thought of my mother, in her final months, terrified when she felt that she was stuck in an unfamiliar subway station, without her bag, not knowing where she was going and who would take her home. "Take me home," you hear echoing in nursing home hallways, and the plaintiveness and the fear and confusion of it, are heartbreaking. You could interpret it as a metaphor for dying itself, or you could interpret it as a basic human need to just go back to all that is familiar and welcoming.

"I have to leave but I can't get out of bed. That's why we're waiting for them to pick us up," Alice cried. She held tightly to my hand with both of hers. I sat on the radiator next to her bed, so I could talk into her good left ear.

Gradually she calmed down. Her grip on my hands loosened. Every once in a while she asked for a sip of water. I brought over a small cup with a straw that had been left on the dresser. She sipped. I stayed with Alice that afternoon until her personal storm passed.

"It's OK to nap," I told her. "I'll be right here."

"I've been napping all afternoon," she snapped, a hint of her feisty self returning, and it made me laugh. She dozed. I caressed her thin hair and told her I'd see her soon.

In his excellent book, *The Best Care Possible,* palliative and hospice pioneer Ira Byock, MD talked about putting up "Get to Know Me" signs in patients' rooms—photos, clippings, mementoes provided by family—so that doctors, nurses and aides would have an idea about who they were caring for. A reminder to treat the ill as the complex, whole people they are. It is a simple, brilliant idea and I wished

Connecting on a Different Plane

there had been signs like that for Flo, Jack and Alice, who I never knew when they were actively engaged in the world, but with whom I tried to connect and comfort.

Leaving the nursing home, I felt exhausted but also pleased that I had been a comfort to Alice. I felt that I'd given her what she needed: I had traveled with her on this dark and frightening part of her journey. I hadn't dismissed her fears or tried to convince her that she was imagining things. Despite the barriers, I felt I had managed to connect with her—on a different plane.

❧❧

Our training curriculum did not include dementia care, which in hindsight seemed like a glaring oversight. According to the Alzheimer's Association, nearly half of the people over the age of 85 have dementia. Life expectancy between diagnosis and death may be eight to 10 years, but 40 percent of that time will be spent in the advanced stage of the illness.

Here's another eye-opener. By the age of 80, only four percent of Americans will enter a nursing home, while 75 percent of those with dementia will do so by the age of 80. Dr. Maribeth Gallagher, dementia program director at Hospice of the Valley in Scottsdale, Arizona, calls it the epidemic of our time.

I've learned about communicating with people with dementia one-on-one, at their bedsides. I've also learned from the passionate experts in the field.

"Individuals with dementia are the most vulnerable

people on the planet," Dr. Carol Long told me. "They can no longer communicate their needs except through behaviors. We see a lot of behaviors of discomfort."

Now a principal of Capstone Healthcare in Phoenix, Arizona, she is renowned for her work with people with dementia. She is best known for her work as program co-director of the palliative care for advanced dementia at the Beatitudes Campus in Phoenix, Arizona. Beatitudes is a nonprofit continuing-care community that partnered with Hospice of the Valley—which had started its own dementia care program in 2003. The program in Scottsdale developed a model of care for people with dementia in 2005. Comfort Matters, Beatitudes' research and education initiative, grew out of that partnership.

Years ago, when people acted out, Dr. Long said, "We believed 'that's who the person is.' Now we believe that the person is uncomfortable and we need to find out the cause of the distress." If someone is hallucinating, for example, and there's no medical reason for it, she said, you provide physical safety and reassure the person that you'll keep him (or her) safe.

Connections are made through a balance of calming and sensory stimulating activities—with hand massage, conversation, flowers, humming songs, for example, and the simple pleasures: reminiscence with memory books or scrapbooks; music therapy, as long as the music represents people's tastes.

Comfort Matters teaches others about providing comfort care for people with advanced dementia. The New York City Chapter of the Alzheimer's Association has been one of

Connecting on a Different Plane

its most ardent followers, bringing the philosophy and practice of comfort care to three large nursing homes in New York. Ann Wyatt, coordinator of the chapter's palliative care project, shared the project's history and findings during a National Provider Call of the Medicare Learning Network. That's a program of the Centers for Medicare and Medicaid Services under its National Partnership to Improve Dementia Care in Nursing Homes. (A transcript of this event is at http://www.cms.gov/Outreach-and-Education/Outreach/NPC/Downloads/2014-12-09-Dementia-Transcript.pdf.)

Among the key points: Behavior is communication. Dementia does not cause the behavior; dementia prevents people from expressing the cause of their distress. Antipsychotic medications may not be responsive to the underlying problem, and may remove the person's only means of communication.

It is as important to know what brings comfort as it is to know what causes distress. Comfort can come from peanut butter sandwiches; chocolate; scrambled eggs; back rubs; the color blue; Frank Sinatra; a walk down the hall; holding hands; pictures of dogs or cats; listening to a baseball game; holding a baby doll; gospel music on an iPod; Bible reading; sitting on a bench outside; a lollipop.

Some call this approach person-centered care. Wyatt, of the Alzheimer's Association, prefers to call it comfort care, a much more concrete term and a way to communicate more easily with family members, nursing home staff, and medical personnel.

"If you can demonstrate that a person with dementia

can be more comfortable, it leads to being more accessible to the family," she told me. "They are more able to feel connected to a person before [that person dies]. And it's better for the staff."

The goal of Wyatt and other dementia-care advocates is to make it the norm to provide palliative care at the time people are diagnosed with the illness. Dr. Maribeth Gallagher stressed that a meeting to talk about goals of care and advance directives should be offered soon after diagnosis and communicated very clearly to those who will make decisions for the person with dementia.

In 2014, Hospice of the Valley was awarded a grant to create a palliative care program for people living with early stages of dementia The program simplified medications, provided caregiver education and four hours of free respite care for caregivers. It featured a crisis phone line for caregivers that was manned by qualified professionals 24 hours a day, seven days a week. The program took note of outcomes, such as hospitalizations and emergency room visits. The result: $369 per member savings per month. Dr. Gallagher believes that the availability of the phone line and skilled professionals to answer calls had the biggest impact on improving outcomes.

"A lot of best practices, like simplifying medications, are affordable," she said. "It's all focused on comfort. People do so much better."

The alternative—the cacophony of a day room with 20 or 30 people in it, residents lashing out verbally and physically at aides, for example—is all too common. As Dr. Gallagher explained, when a brain is not engaged, and not able to

Connecting on a Different Plane

process information conventionally, it defaults to what it can do, which leads to hypervigilance and mounting anxiety. The solution, in her words, is to "make the brain a better offer." This entails engaging with a sensory experience, or even offering something as simple, soothing and satisfying as chocolate.

5

Unfinished Business

In hospice training, we talked about the Big Questions that people often focus on close to the end of their lives, if they are blessed with a clear, conscious mind: What did my life mean? Why was I here? What was my purpose? What is my legacy?

Despite ample evidence to the contrary, I do believe in the possibility—and the importance—of resolution, reconciliation, and redemption.

But for Bobby and for Jane, there was none of that, and I couldn't seem to make it better.

I felt anxious on my way to meet Bobby for the first time, not only because I'm directionally challenged, but also because he was the first person I visited who was my age.

Last Comforts

Most people I visit are my senior by at least 20 years or more. So this was too close to home, you might say; a reminder that, yes, it can happen to you. Worse, he was in hospice care for ALS (amyotrophic lateral sclerosis, or Lou Gehrig's disease). I had encountered the cruel impact of ALS with my aunt 15 years earlier.

ALS is a relatively rare illness, afflicting roughly two people per 100,000 per year, according to the Robert Packard Center for ALS at Johns Hopkins. The ALS Association reports that 5,600 people in the U.S. are diagnosed with ALS each year and that as many as 30,000 Americans may have the disease at any given time. About half of patients live at least two years after diagnosis; 20 percent live five years or more and up to 10 percent survive more than 10 years.

I wound my way through quiet streets in the kind of neighborhood where the only people you see during the day are landscapers, contractors and housecleaning services and where one house is grander than the next. I felt anxious as I pulled up to the home of Bobby's brother and sister-in-law. Bobby had been staying in their large brick ranch house since the diagnosis. As his contemporary, I was thinking that maybe Bobby and I would have a lot in common: growing up in the '60s, the music, the culture, all of that. Maybe we could get to be real friends.

Bobby's Filipino aide, Linda, opened the front door and led me from the light and airy foyer to a dark and cluttered family room that felt like a cave with a large screen TV and a stereo system. The house was silent. No one had turned on any lamps. Bobby, sitting in one of three wheelchairs positioned side by side, greeted me with a wan handshake. He was heavy and pear-shaped, with a full head of gray-white hair and lopsided glasses.

Linda stayed in the corner of the room. Bobby repeatedly asked for her help in shifting from one wheelchair to another to adjust his head. The disease had already sapped the strength he needed to control his neck. She also gave him sips of water when he called out to her, which was often.

That first meeting was as awkward as a blind date. We traded condensed versions of our bios. He told me about his sporting goods store; and how rollerblading in Central Park used to be his favorite thing. He wished he could do that again. He was angry about the diagnosis, angry about how doctors in two different hospitals explained—insensitively and yelling, in one case, he said—that the disease was incurable.

Just before I left, he said in a voice weakened by illness, "There's no hope."

"All I want is a cure."

I felt I couldn't leave without responding, that he needed his fear and despair acknowledged.

"Well, there's a different kind of hope," I said. Even though this is what I truly believe—that there can be hope for good days, for good companionship, for the comfort of being with friends or family, for seeing another season—my words sounded hollow even to me.

I visited Bobby once or twice a week for several months that spring. We had little in common. He liked movies, but his taste ran to thrillers and the Godfather series, not indies or classics. He had not been a Beatles or Rolling Stones fan in the '60s. He liked Howard Stern and the misogynistic comedian Andrew Dice Clay. He messed up in school, never went to college, did not marry or have kids. He brightened only in talking about his three German shepherds that he missed so much. They remained in his house in a nearby town, cared for by his girlfriend Jenny.

"Can't the dogs stay here? Or visit?" I asked one day. He looked at me as if I'd asked if he could leap out of the chair and fly away.

"No," he said. "My brother hates dogs. He's very strict."

❧❧

"Guess how much this wheelchair cost?" Bobby asked me one unexpectedly warm day in early April when he and Linda were sitting outside on the wide front patio to greet me.

"I don't know. $5,000?" I said, as I sat down on the patio's low wall, to join them.

"Hah!" He cast a knowing glance at Linda. He was almost gleeful. This plush motorized chair's controls were easy enough for him to manage without assistance; he practically did twirls for me. The chair still had a tag with his name on it, like a new car. It looked like it could do anything but make your morning coffee.

So I guessed a few more times, rising in $5,000 increments until I hit $25,000.

"Right!"

"Wow! That's more than my Camry cost," I said. That

was the appalling truth. I wondered how are they paying for it? Does insurance cover the chair? What do people do if they can't afford these things?

One time he asked Linda to scratch his face. He couldn't do that for himself.

"I can't even feed myself anymore," he wailed.

What would it be like to have an itch and not be able to scratch it? It sounded like such a miniscule thing, compared to the tsunami of destruction that is ALS. But I couldn't help thinking about that, and about being confined to a chair, or a bed, increasingly unable to move, to breathe, to talk, or to swallow. Even if you were a person who'd always lived so much in your head, your gorgeous mind romping happily wherever it chose, glad to spend hours on end being nourished by books and magazines and music and movies, would that be enough to compensate for the loss of your physical self? Would that corrode your soul? Would you succumb to despair? Would you go mad?

While life may be short, the boredom of illness can stretch a day immeasurably. Bobby had no interest in reading, felt that he had watched all there was to watch on TV, didn't want to do much of anything. Certainly he didn't want to write—or dictate—his life story for his nieces and nephews, with whom he felt he had nothing in common. His main goal, which seemed increasingly elusive, was to have a stair lift installed in his own house, so he could return there to live.

Last Comforts

I wanted to find something to engage Bobby, to help him break out of his despair, fear, and depression. In short, I wanted to make things better. I found a telephone support group for ALS patients and their families, and called his brother to suggest Bobby try it: Wednesdays, 3 pm, for an hour. Much to my surprise, he actually did call in—though he found it too depressing.

"One guy talked about planning his own funeral," he said, horrified.

"You know, maybe he felt like that would give him some kind of control back, over his life," I replied, but Bobby wasn't buying it. I changed the subject. I noticed he was using a neck brace for support. The back of the chair he was in that afternoon wasn't high enough.

"There are gadgets for everything," I said, talking about the brace and thinking that my aunt probably could have used one of these things.

"I hate 'em all," he said.

When I left that day, I asked if he'd like me to bring him more diet chocolate ice cream from the local ice cream parlor he favored. Or if there was anything else I could do.

"I wish you could tell me there's a cure," he said.

"I wish I could too."

I brought a checkers set with me the week after he told me he liked playing checkers. He seemed pleased that I remembered. I won the first game we played. By the time we played the second game, he didn't have the strength to move his own pieces, but indicated to me where they should go. He won that game, which annoyed me no end.

"Two out of three?" I asked, my competitive streak rearing its sly little head. But he was too tired.

Another time, when his voice was giving out, I told him I could play some music on my iPhone with the Pandora music app.

"Can you get Johnny Cash?" he asked. And I did, cranking up the volume. We sat in comfortable silence, me on the couch in the dimly lit family room, Bobby in one of the wheelchairs, as Johnny croaked about Folsom Prison and being caught in a ring of fire.

Bobby was released from his own prison in early May, which I learned via email from our volunteer coordinator. Just a few days before he died, I'd met Jenny and her high school-age daughter Halley, who came by for a little while. I told Bobby a joke that my granddaughter had told me: what kind of karate move does a pig have? A pork chop. Haha.

"Jenny, come in, you have to hear this joke," he called out; Jenny and Linda were sisters-in-law and they were in the kitchen, catching up and laughing at jokes of their own. It was the first time I'd actually heard Linda laughing.

Jenny was outgoing and affectionate with Bobby. The week before, he had said that when he told her she'd have to go on after he was gone, she didn't want to hear it.

"She pretends there'll be a cure even more than I do," he told me.

After Jenny and Halley left, another friend showed up and presented Bobby with a large, detailed drawing of his three dogs. "You can't have the dogs here, but at least you can look at their picture," she said. After a few pleasantries I left, not wanting to tire him out more and letting them have some time together.

"You can stay," he said to me, but I told him, "No, I'll let you two visit and I'll call you Monday, OK?"

That was where we left it.

Later, I thought about how he left the world, in anxiety and in fear, with so many regrets.

"I should have fixed up my house."

"I wouldn't have gained and lost the weight so many times."

"I should have sold the business. I stayed in it too long."

His despair was inordinately sad. What did I do? I was just a visitor, who played some checkers, played some music, told jokes, and listened to him expressing his fears, his anger, and his sadness without telling him everything was going to be OK.

A witness.

Jane

Jane was not a lucky woman. She'd been married, but her husband died in his late 40s, not long after they adopted their second daughter. Although she was not a smoker, Jane had lung cancer that spread "everywhere except to the heart," as she explained to me the first time I visited at her tidy, modest home near the New Jersey Meadowlands. She'd been an accountant until her "forced retirement," as she called it. Jane entered hospice care after a surgeon recommended an above-knee amputation because the cancer had invaded her thigh. She replied, 'No. Enough is enough.'

"They gave me a three-month prognosis," she said, matter-of-factly, during that first visit. "It really messes with your head, just waiting to die."

Jane couldn't afford to sit and wait. With a full "to do" list, Jane methodically began taking care of countless details that had to be attended to, mostly involving her high school-age daughters, the elder of whom was headed to college in the fall. She did this from her living room couch, which was moved to the corner of the room to accommodate a hospital bed that she, so far, refused to use. She wanted to set up a trust for them. She wanted to find scholarship money for Julie, her older daughter, for college. She wanted to finish her income taxes. Someone from her church asked her if she'd begun "farewell letters" to her children, but she had not. There were other priorities too.

She told me she lived from one milestone to the next: she was alive for her own birthday; next, she was aiming for Julie's 18th birthday the following month.

"It's all you can do," I said. "It's all any of us can do, really."

"I don't know where my kids are going to live," she said, getting suddenly teary. Her husband's family was not an option. Neither was her sister, who had already said she wouldn't give up smoking even if that meant not being able to open her home to Julie and to Danielle, who is asthmatic.

Last Comforts

Jane's "official" caregiver was her aunt Patty, in her late 70s, who lived an hour away and had health issues of her own, so she was not available either.

Jane's nurse case manager had asked for a volunteer for Jane ostensibly because, in the afternoons, she was lonely and had no one to talk to. By that time in my volunteering experience, I didn't necessarily expect to be the sole visitor in a household and indeed, during the course of a two-hour visit, Aunt Patty and Jane's minister and her sister and cousin came by too.

It was all fairly easy-going and convivial, until Danielle came home from school. It was like a stage entrance by a character full of anger and negative energy, as if she was in mid-argument with someone, or possibly, with herself. Without greeting Jane, she headed straight for the computer set up in the dining area and started in mid-sentence: "I need to use your computer. I have a paper on food that's due tomorrow." She sat down noisily at the desk and kept coughing. Jane sternly asked her to please put on a mask if the coughing continued because Jane couldn't afford to catch anything right now. Danielle snatched a mask from the side table next to Jane and returned to the computer.

I wondered if the girls were getting any kind of counseling. They were probably angry with Jane for being sick and dying. And scared. And wondering what their life was going to be like, afterward. Jane told me that Julie, in a rare reflective moment, had recently asked her, "Who will walk me down the aisle?"

Not surprisingly, the girls were self-absorbed and foul.

Unfinished Business

I wondered how they would feel in five, ten, or twenty years. Would they still be angry or filled with regret? Would they continue to be resentful that fate dealt them an awful hand? Or, would they thrive in a new life, having shed the old like a snake sheds its skin?

I made a point of going over to Danielle to say goodbye when it was time to leave, wishing her luck with her paper. Wanly, she shook my hand. In the car, I used hand sanitizer because I too did not want to catch her cold.

❧❧

Conversations with Jane meandered. We rarely dwelled on the elephant in the room. We shared recipes for soups. She told me about a sauerkraut soup that uses lima beans cooked and blended (an odd combination, but she said it was delicious) and at the end, a roux of butter and flour to thicken it. I told her about the hearty Portuguese cabbage, leek, and carrot soup recipe I'd gotten during a vacation in Portugal. She recalled fondly a great roast beef sandwich at an old place in a nearby town, where she'd gone with her father, and pastries from a local Polish bakery. It's the small pleasures that stay with us until the end, it seems.

One time an old friend visited Jane for a few days. They crafted a letter for Jane to sign, allowing teachers to call local friends in the event that Jane couldn't talk on the phone. Jane was also on the phone trying to reach her nurse about her pain medications. Jane experienced major pain the night before, but didn't want morphine because she didn't like the way it made her feel. She'd taken other pills but those weren't helping. Exhausted, she finally fell back to sleep around six in the morning.

One of the great benefits of hospice care is that help is available any time, seven days a week. Had the nurse case manager and social worker not explained that? Or, had Jane simply not heard it? Palliative and hospice doctors and nurses always stress that there is never a reason for a person to be in pain. If there's "breakthrough" pain, it can be addressed day or night.

I gave Jane's friend the main hospital number to call after hours and told her to ask for the hospice-nurse case manager on call, suggesting that if Jane had another night like the one before, she had to call for help. She wrote down the information and put it up on the refrigerator.

Jane assigned her friend the task of going to the bank to find out if she could get into Jane's safe deposit box, so Jane could weed what she didn't need. She also planned to go through her jewelry that night, to figure out who would get what.

When Danielle came home that day, she seemed genuinely glad to see Jane's friend, and said a quick hello before trotting upstairs. But she still didn't greet Jane.

Soon afterward, our volunteer coordinator called to let me know that Jane was transferred to Holy Name Medical Center as a GIP (General In-Patient) and that she'd let me know if she learned anything further. Shortly after that, Jane went to Holy Name's freestanding 20-bed hospice Villa Marie Claire in Saddle River, so they could get her pain medications right and give the family the chance to find someone to live

Unfinished Business

in with her 24/7 upon her return home.

I visited Jane at Villa Marie Claire. She was sound asleep in her room. I greeted her but there was no response. Her glasses were off and she wasn't on oxygen. She looked amazingly peaceful. Her cell phone, resting on the rolling table by her bedside, rang a number of times and she didn't stir.

I stayed an hour, which felt meditative. It's very quiet at Villa Marie Claire. There isn't the noise and bustle of a nursing home or a hospital and the view of the expansive lawn and distant trees, even on this cold first day of spring, was soothing. An aide came by to put a pillow under Jane's arm, which had dropped over the side of the bed. Even that didn't wake her.

Jane was still at Villa Marie Claire a week later. Her bed had been repositioned so she was right by the window, with a picture of her and her daughters on the windowsill. She awakened briefly when I came in and said hello, and then fell back to sleep.

A nurse came in to give Jane medication. One of the reasons I love these nurses is that they treat patients with affection and respect no matter their condition. The nurse explained to Jane everything she was about to do, what she was doing as she was doing it, and fluffed up the pillow before she left.

Sometimes I think I volunteer to wrap my head around the idea of mortality—my own, in particular—but I think the truth is, it feels impossible. I can no sooner fathom what Jane had been going through—was going through then—than I can envision walking on the moon. It seemed to me that her anguish may have already been behind her; all those details, all those preparations, all that unfinished business, whatever messages/love/words of wisdom she may have wanted to share with her daughters, all past now. She was past that.

The gift Jane gave to her elder daughter Julie was that she did not die on Julie's birthday, so at least Julie won't have that extra-added burden in her life. I called Aunt Patty, but could only leave a message on her voicemail and I never heard back from her. It's a peculiar thing to be a volunteer, landing in the midst of someone's life, and then, whoosh, flying back out of it again. I'll probably never know how the lives of Julie and Danielle will evolve. The last couple of months had been a short, incomplete story with no resolution, not unlike the end of Jane's life.

The postscript: Twice a year Holy Name holds a memorial service for the families of people who have died during the previous six months. Several months after Jane died, I attended the service and, not seeing anyone connected with Jane, asked one of the bereavement counselors about the family. They didn't know anything either; the home phone had been disconnected and letters of condolence had been returned, addressee unknown. They could never reach Aunt Patty either. I did find the girls on Facebook and it looks like their lives are proceeding (which I mentioned to the bereavement counselors). I did not message them. And so, the story remains unresolved.

6

I've Got All My Sisters With Me

It was Wednesday afternoon before Thanksgiving, and I found myself in the unlikely position of standing before a group of about two dozen retired nuns, reciting Hebrew prayers for Chanukah, because that night would be the first night of the holiday. As the rock group Talking Heads used to sing, how did I get here?

For a happy period of volunteering one fall and early winter, I was assigned to visit two retired nuns at St. Michael Villa, a stunning Romanesque Revival building atop the Palisades in Englewood Cliffs, New Jersey. With breathtaking views of the Hudson River and George Washington Bridge, the villa, built as a novitiate in 1938 by the Sisters of St. Joseph of Peace, was now a home where elder nuns were cared for. The Sisters of St. Joseph of Peace founded Holy Name Hospital in 1925.

Last Comforts

Although technically I was there to visit Sister S and Sister N, I quickly became part of a group of eight to a dozen nuns who gathered in mid-morning with activities director Norma for exercise, iced tea, listening to music, art, or game playing. Some of the nuns had dementia; some were recovering from strokes. Most were either in wheelchairs or walked with a walker. Norma, incredibly creative in coming up with arts projects and games, was affectionate and patient with the nuns, teasing them and encouraging them to do just another leg lift, just one more series of arm circles.

Each Sister had her own room; the rooms were spare but light-filled and clean and offered calming views of the surrounding greenery or the spectacular Hudson River and upper Manhattan. The villa was filled with numerous public spaces, including an activities room, a main gathering space, and a dining area where meals were served with cloth napkins and tablecloths. Another large dining hall and a chapel were downstairs.

After only a few visits, the nuns accepted me with warmth and affection. On warmer fall days, I joined the group outdoors on the terrace to soak up the sun, the view, and the tranquility. Sister B, in her 90s, was elfin, always ready to get up and help distribute apple juice and cookies, or organize materials for arts and crafts, always quick with a joke.

She was the one who told me about how Sister S had been a social worker that she'd met while Sister B worked at an orphanage. She pressed her head to Sister S's. Then she'd cup her head in her hands, and say, "Remember how the

I've Got All My Sisters with Me

children sang 'Here comes Sister S, flying through the air.'" Sister S responded with a slight smile. Sister S didn't communicate conventionally. When she spoke, which wasn't often, I couldn't make out what she was saying, except once. When Norma played an audiotape in the common room, Sister S sang along with "How Great Thou Art," all the verses, loud and clear.

While it was still warm enough to sit outside, Sister B spoke to Sister S, who did not respond. With great tenderness, Sister B turned to me and said, "She's in another world now."

While Sister S was sweet and gentle, Sister N. was not. Though she couldn't talk, Sister N was a formidable presence—she could gaze at you so intensely, you wondered what she was seeing and thinking. She could look alarmed, or fearful. Sometimes, when she was wheeled outside the activities room, seated with a few other wheelchair-bound nuns, her eyes, her face, seemed at peace.

The nursing coordinator at St. Michael's once told me that Sister N had been the nurse who had trained her. One day I told Sister N about how kind a nun had been the day my then two-year-old son was in the hospital for stitches in his forehead, after another child had pushed a swing into his head at the playground. My husband took care of our son that day; I was out doing an interview for the weekly housing column I wrote for The New York Times.

This was before the advent of cell phones. When I got home and got the message that they were at the hospital I raced over and found the room where my son's deep

89

cut was being stitched. For some reason, I had to stay in the hall, though, and I paced back and forth listening to my son screaming—feeling a storm of worry, pain, and guilt (for not being with him at the park). A nun walking by, stopped and said to me, "The time you have to worry is when they're quiet."

It was a moment of real kindness, and it calmed me. Could it have been Sister N? If this were a movie, it would have been, but in reality? Probably not. But telling her about the memory was my way of thanking whoever it was that calmed me during that stressful time.

One week, I sat next to Sister N as we all, in a circle, played "parachute." You've probably seen this in pre-schools. The parachute is a big, colorful circle of plastic that we all took hold of (those of us who could) and then flapped it up and down to bounce balls on top of it. Then Norma or I, or sometimes Sister B, chased the balls that inevitably bounced over the parachute. You could see a glimmer of pleasure on Sister N's face, as if she were thinking, well this is ridiculous but kind of fun. It made Sister W—once a Mother Superior—smile her big toothless grin (as did the large bubbles that Norma blew in good weather out on the terrace).

Meanwhile, Sister C was off by herself at the art table, in the common area, but not too far from everyone else. She suffered from dementia and liked to spend her time drawing, or coloring in the many pictures that Norma had collected for them. Sister C liked the color green in particular. Once she colored in a paper that had the word "Peace" printed on it. And this is what she wrote on her own in the margins: "Life

I've Got All My Sisters with Me

is a river that flows all around us setting the darkness free."

Sometimes I spent time alone with Sister N and Sister S, but mostly we were together as a group until it was time to wheel them into the dining room for lunch.

As fall wore on, Norma and I talked about how odd it was that this year, Chanukah and Thanksgiving fell on the same day. Then Norma, also Jewish, had her brainstorm: why not do a presentation to the nuns about Chanukah, the day before Thanksgiving? We could do it together, she said.

And that is how I found myself, on that Wednesday afternoon, helping Norma decorate the common room with paper menorahs and dreidels, pouring wine into small cups to distribute later, and setting out trays of jelly doughnuts and gold, coin-shaped chocolates (Chanukah gelt) that Norma brought. We greeted a group of about two dozen retired nuns after lunch that day, and began the presentation by lighting the menorah I brought from home and saying the Hebrew prayer for it.

I spoke briefly about why we celebrate Chanukah—the story of a courageous and successful rebellion against religious oppression. Then I lifted a glass of wine and said the Hebrew blessing. We sang songs. We gave the nuns—those who remained awake—jelly doughnuts and small cups of wine. Some took turns playing the dreidel game, rewarded with chocolate "coins" if they won.

But, the biggest hit was the "pin the candle on the menorah" game that Norma had set up, hanging the menorah on a column in the room. Several of our morning group took part, while others rooted for them, shouting "warmer...

Last Comforts

warmer," as they got closer to the menorah; or "colder...
colder," as they moved farther from the target. It was silly. It
was fun. It was less than educational. More than a few would
remember little about it though I was glad we did it. "God
bless you," one of the nuns said to me, as I cleaned up afterward. We hugged.

In early winter, one morning Norma started exercise
time by asking each Sister what exercise the group should do.
Sister D, recovering from a stroke, said "I had a bad dream
and it's called exercise." Later that morning, she told a fairly long story—the most I'd heard her speak since I'd been
here—about the time decades earlier, how she was here doing
spring cleaning, at the building that stood on this site before it burned down. When the fire started, the nuns asked
a young boy to call the police; it was April 1 and he was a
child. The police didn't believe him and the building burned
down. Sister B recalled another Sister whisking one child out
of a bathtub to safety.

Close to Christmas, while Norma was called away
from the group to take a call, she handed me the sheets of
daily tidbits she shared with the group. That day it was all
about Christmas. I got to an item about Dec. 26 being St.
Stephen's Day. It was also referred to as Boxing Day, having
to do with the first Christian martyr. But it had nothing at all
to do with boxing or horse racing. Sister B began singing a
little song that, as she explained, she and other children went
from house to house singing, in effect, asking for a treat. This
was in Ireland.

I've Got All My Sisters with Me

Sister L sang it too. Sister G, sitting next to me, was amazed that Sister L remembered this. And then, Sister G told me about how her mother always had treats on hand for the children, because it was so important to share. They didn't have much, she said, but her mother always told her, "It's the little things that count."

Indeed they do.

I always felt at peace when leaving St. Michael's. When I tried to analyze why that was so, I thought, there is peace in community. We are social creatures, after all. And maybe it's a great comfort to be side-by-side with your sisters even if you cannot communicate with them, or you don't remember the day, the hour, or the minute before.

Our lives are so much richer when we connect with our friends and our families and remain socially engaged. When serious illness strikes, wouldn't it be a comfort not to lose those connections? Wouldn't it be better not to live in isolation, whether it's in a nursing home or even in one's own home attended by caregivers and aides?

Granted, the Sisters had long been accustomed to living in community. A life of faith had given them a strong foundation to withstand losses, personal or otherwise, or to bear the loss of companionship when one or another died. But there was something about this home that was nurturing even for those who couldn't speak, or sing, or draw, or do seated exercises, or who spent much of their time asleep, but remained in the midst of the group.

In the months I spent visiting St. Michael's, I never heard the plaintive, agitated, or angry cries so common in nursing homes. The nuns accepted each other as they were and found comfort in each other's company. The rhythm of their days was prescribed, but peaceful and predictable. Could this be replicated in a secular environment? As I learned much later, the short answer is yes, and I'll tell you more about that in Chapter 11.

Part Two

7

Reality TV

A li MacGraw's Disease: Movie illness in which the only symptom is that the sufferer grows more beautiful as death approaches. —Roger Ebert, "Glossary of Movie Terms" (Abridged)

Why are we so hesitant to talk about mortality, or to recognize it, when it is right there in front of us, in plain sight? Let's look at our popular culture, because it's such a potent factor in both reflecting and shaping our attitudes about life and death. Though our movies, television, and video games may be awash in hideous, sudden, and violent deaths, it is extremely rare to see what it really looks like to die.

For decades, Hollywood has given us what the late film critic Roger Ebert called movie disease, where dying never seems to diminish a character's camera-ready looks, independence or eloquence. I'm a fan of the weepie genre

Last Comforts

as much as anyone and my award for best movie death goes to *Dark Victory,* from 1939. It stars Bette Davis as a spoiled party-girl heiress who finds deeper meaning in life after she's been diagnosed with a terminal brain tumor (and marries her surgeon, to boot).

We learn, as does Bette, that once her eyesight goes, she will die soon after. So here's what happens: Now happily married, she is spending an idyllic afternoon gardening with her good and devoted friend, played by Geraldine Fitzgerald, in the Vermont home she shares with her husband. He is preparing to leave for a medical conference. She comments to Geraldine how odd it is that the weather is so warm, considering how it has gotten to be so cloudy. Ooops! She realizes what is happening. As her eyesight fails, she manages to find her way upstairs and convinces her husband to go alone to the conference. After he leaves, she lies down on her bed, ever so decorously, and dies quickly, quietly, and peacefully.

I understand the need to take artistic license. Within the context of a two-hour film, it's hard to convey a slow decline that has its ups and downs over a period of time, the almost infinite number of ways the body's functions break down and become unpredictable, not to mention the times spent uncommunicative either because of fatigue, weakness, and deep sleep or declining cognitive function. Showing the slow progression also would not be particularly dramatic, uplifting, or satisfying to the audience. But, having been with my mother, and others since, grappling with the nasty effects of a brain tumor, I can say that Bette's experience is pretty close to a fairy tale.

Reality TV

Fast forward 40 years. In 1970, the blockbuster *Love Story,* based on Erich Segal's bestselling book, told the tale of the doomed love of Oliver and Jenny (played by Ryan O'Neal and Ali MacGraw). After a storybook college romance and post-graduation marriage, Jenny is diagnosed with a terminal disease, which is never specified, though we may assume it is cancer. At the end, from her hospital bed, where she lays decorously, she makes her own funeral arrangements with her father's help and then asks to see Oliver. They share a final embrace and she quietly dies.

In 1988, we had *Beaches,* an old-fashioned weepie about the friendship between two wildly different women (Barbara Hershey, whose character comes from an aristocratic background and Bette Midler, in a caricature of her persona as a headstrong, flamboyant Jewish singer/actor). Bette takes care of Barbara after Barbara is diagnosed with movie disease.

Her diagnosis is fleetingly specified as viral endocarditis, a heart ailment. As her illness progresses, her makeup does make her look pallid, though her hair always looks great. Except for a short period in which she languishes in pajamas until Bette upbraids her for it, she dresses well too. When Barbara collapses and is hospitalized, Bette rushes to her side and next thing we know, Bette manages to spirit Barbara out of the hospital because Barbara doesn't want her daughter to see her there. They repair to Barbara's beach house. Our last view of Barbara is from the rear, as the two friends sit decorously on deck chairs with the sun rapidly and symbolically setting in the distance. We might presume that Barbara dies quickly, quietly, and peacefully for we never see her final moments.

Last Comforts

Television may give us fewer movie deaths, but it provides many more heroic moments of back-from-the-brink, life-saving measures. One of my favorite medical studies, published in the *New England Journal of Medicine* in June 1996, showed that TV portrayals of cardiopulmonary resuscitation are dramatically more successful than in real life. They are misleading in several major ways that can easily lead to a viewer's misunderstanding its considerable risks.

Here's what the researchers did. Dr. Susan Diem of Durham VA Medical Center, Dr. James Tulsky of Duke University Medical Center, and Dr. John D. Lantos of the University of Chicago viewed a total of 97 episodes of *Chicago Hope, ER,* and *Rescue 911* during the 1994-5 season. They and recorded the patients' sex and age; location, cause, and number of cardiac arrests; who performed the CPR; survival rates and long-term outcomes; and number of deaths. As if that wasn't enough, two independent, board-certified internists validated the coding methods by viewing samples of each show and recording data in accordance with the guidelines established for the study.

Here's what they found: 77 percent of patients receiving CPR on *Chicago Hope, ER,* and *Rescue 911* survived their immediate cardiac arrest. The TV patients were overwhelmingly young, healthy victims of gunshot wounds, car wrecks, or similar traumatic injuries. All but one patient survived cardiac arrest with no long-term disability.

In reality, the majority of people receiving CPR are elderly or hospitalized patients with heart disease, cancer, or other chronic conditions. Among those who survive the initial resuscitation, many die shortly afterward or suffer permanent neurological damage caused by their disease or by the rescue effort itself, the researchers emphasized.

Survival for real-life patients, they said, ranges from 2 percent to 30 percent for out-of-hospital cardiac arrests and 6.5 percent to 15 percent for in-hospital arrests. For trauma cardiac arrests, survival rates vary from one percent to 30 percent, depending on the type of injury. The study also found that most TV patients either fully recovered or immediately died after CPR, excluding a third possibility of long-term or permanent disability caused by their disease or the CPR itself.

Veering from reality for the sake of art could be forgiven if it didn't have potentially harmful consequences. If you're thinking about drafting your advance directive and considering whether you'd want CPR, you might make a different decision if you had an overly optimistic view of the technique's likely success, based on what you've seen on television.

I wish that we had the equivalent of the GLAAD media awards. Every year since 1990, GLAAD, the lesbian, gay, bisexual and transgender (LGBT) media advocacy organization, has awarded films, television series, and feature stories for excellence in exploring LGBT issues. It has become quite the star-studded affair. It is broadcast on cable television, and generates a tidal wave of publicity.

Right now, if we did have a similar awards event for accurate portrayal about late life, to whom would those awards go? Alas, few recent films and TV programs might qualify, with the notable exceptions of *Still Alice,* about a professor diagnosed with early-onset Alzheimer's disease, and the documentary *Alive Inside,* about the remarkable power of music—specifically, individualized playlists based on people's own favorites—to comfort those with dementia. [1] Another notable exception is *Life Itself,* based on Roger Ebert's autobiography of the same name—a documentary that looks unflinchingly at the critic's struggles at the end of his life and celebrates the great love he and his wife Chaz shared.

What do people look like when they're close to death? What's the reality of caring for loved ones in decline? We're not likely to see the rawness, the intimacy, the messiness, the profundity of it on TV. Or, at least, we weren't, until Magical Elves, a company that also brings us *Top Chef* and *Project Runway,* produced an extraordinary six-part documentary that aired in 2013 on the Showtime network. It was called *Time of Death.*

The series originated with an idea by co-executive producer Miggi Hood to do a show about families coming together over a loved one's deathbed. It was based on insights Hood had come to about conflict and reconciliation during her mother's last days. It was originally titled, *Dying to See You.* For two years, Hood researched death and dying and interviewed people who had experienced loss. In August 2012, Magical Elves showed some of these interviews to Showtime, which ordered the series. By then it had morphed into a series about people and their families facing the final months, weeks, and days before death.

The six-part series showed a cross-section of people ranging in age from 19 to 78, who were of diverse genders, races, and religions. Some were in a good place emotionally and spiritually at the time of death while others struggled to come to terms with their complicated lives. In all, the series focused on eight people and their families. I came to love all of them.

The series raised many questions for me: How had Magical Elves found these remarkably courageous people and their families? Why did they agree to be filmed up to and, in some cases, including the very end? How did the film company make the leap from food, fashion and pop culture into what is truly reality TV? Would the series find a second life as a training tool for physicians, nurses, social workers, and community groups? I contacted co-producer Alexandra Lipsitz to find out.

She told me it took a year and a half to find people. The search included outreach to hospice groups, the medical community, and social media. Filming involved small crews where the producers were the camera operators and confidantes of the family and the ill. Participants signed a Health Insurance Portability and Accountability Act (HIPAA) waiver, which was necessary because protecting patient privacy under HIPAA is paramount. Ordinarily, real names, medical details, and treatments cannot be divulged publicly.

Throughout the course of filming, the producers depended on hospice and other health-care professionals to provide insight into the dying process and to prepare them for what was to come. One hospice worker, featured in the series, came to Magical Elves' offices regularly to counsel the producers and editors working on the show because the experience was so intense for all.

Last Comforts

The producers visited some people over a few days' time; others were filmed over a longer period. Sometimes they filmed around the clock. The families were clear about what they wanted to share—and what they didn't. Usually, Lipsitz explained, she has other people doing camera work. This time, she shot much of the series herself.

"We were pretty honest in the outreach process," Lipsitz told me. When she visited people, she brought her camera, to give them a sense of what filming would be like. Single parent Maria, 48, a fiercely independent woman struggling with stage 4 breast cancer, was the first person she met. Lipsitz recalled that Maria asked, "You mean there's going to be a camera up my butt?"

In fact, the series focuses much of its attention on Maria—whom Lipsitz admired for her warrior attitude, her humor, and her devotion to her children even when she was yelling at them. Daughter Nicole (nicknamed "Little") was in her mid-twenties. Her two teen children (and Little's half-siblings) were Julia and Andrew.

Maria's goal was to see Little become guardian of the teens after her death, rather than her ex-husband. Throughout filming, she tries whatever treatment she could to stay alive long enough to see that happen. Julia and Andrew, being teens, behave badly, express their anger freely, and are not at all sure they want to live with Little. Their rage and sullenness was so like what I had seen with Jane and her daughters, Julie and Danielle in Chapter 5, I wanted to reach through the TV screen to shake them by their shoulders and say, Pay attention, and cherish this brief time you have with your mother!

Reality TV

Of course, they must grapple with grief in their own way.

For a time, Julia and Andrew go to foster care. In the meantime, Maria's condition declines as her cancer spreads and impairs her mentally and emotionally. The camera follows Little as she finds Maria, dead in her bed at home.

It is heart wrenching.

As for the idea that it might be considered a little odd for a company, which had not previously had any exposure to palliative and hospice care, to tackle this subject, Lipsitz said the company founders—her sister Jane Lipsitz and Dan Cutforth—and their crew are "very versatile. They bring thoughtfulness, respect, and reverence to it. I think you can do any subject with grace, dignity, and creativity."

Why did people open up their lives and their homes to Magical Elves? Each had his or her reasons. Families wanted to share how remarkable their loved ones were; those who were dying wanted to make their end meaningful, or to help others who are experiencing the same thing. People also wanted to be remembered. That was certainly the case with Lenore, 75, who said she wanted to do this as the final exploration in her 40 years of work as a psychotherapist in the field of death and dying. She did not want aggressive treatment for her inoperable pancreatic cancer because she had seen first-hand how devastating that kind of treatment can be not only for a patient, but for the patient's family as well.

Lenore's story was moving because of her clarity about what she wanted to do; and also because it showed how reconciliation and healing can take place in a family even if one person is at the end of her life. One of her sons, who had had a troubled and complex adult life, devoted much of his time to caring for his mother at the end. As a result, he found inner strength and maturity.

Reconciliation came to Cheyenne, too, a 47-year-old former mixed martial arts fighter who had been diagnosed with ALS in 2009. Although he was paralyzed and could speak only through a computerized voice he controlled with his eye, Cheyenne was emotionally expressive and had what Lipsitz, the co-producer, called a devilish smile. Long estranged from his mother, the camera captures their reunion, as well as the reunion that his mother subsequently engineered with Cheyenne's two sons, whom he did not know. By the time he died, Cheyenne experienced the love and family support that had eluded him for years.

The families may have been initially wary about being filmed, Lipsitz said, but after a few visits or sometimes, only hours, the producers were embraced as friends or family members.

When 19-year-old Nicolle Kissee was dying of advanced stage melanoma, Nicolle's father and relatives prayed over her and sang. Lipsitz saw a feeling of acceptance on Nicolle's face. "I teared up. I felt overcome," she said. Another "goosebumps" moment came when 78-year-old Morris "Brad" Bradley Jr., a 22-year career military veteran who was suffering from congenital heart failure, told his wife Verda and their daughters that he was resigned to death, that he had made his peace with it and was ready to go. Later, his family told Lipsitz that they were grateful for what they had done,

Reality TV

because Brad never would have said these things except that he was being filmed.

I asked Lipsitz how working on this series affected her. "It was challenging on so many levels," she said. "But what we were going through was nothing compared to the people we were filming.

"You're a human being first and a film crew second," she added. "Maria knew my two-year-old daughter. Lenore too. I'm still in contact with Little and her brother and sister. And all the crew went to visit the Kissee family; we got Christmas cookies from them."

She said she had never before been present when anyone passed away, so she had to confront that. In the course of working on the series, the Lipsitz's stepbrother died of cancer, which "made it all the more real. I became more empathetic. I've given more thought to how I want to live my life."

She also found that "there's so much healing in listening. People want to be heard." And she "learned how important it is to show up when people are alive as well as when they're dying and not to forget to be with whoever is grieving afterwards."

After filming the series was complete, Lipsitz made a conscious choice to take five months off, mainly to spend time with her then-two-year-old daughter.

What did the producers hope to achieve at the end of the series? They wanted to help start a conversation, for people to talk to their family members and friends about how they think and feel about death; and about their fears too. Most important, they hoped that people would think more about what is important to them, to take a moment, and not to take anything for granted.

Time of Death received a modicum of publicity and press coverage, but never became the subject of the kind of "water cooler" public discussion that shows like Homeland or Breaking Bad have. It aired on Friday nights, which may have had something to do with that, although it was (and still is, at this writing) available on demand on the Showtime website. It is not available on DVD or for streaming. And, no, it is not being promoted as a teaching tool.

Video as Teaching Tool on YouTube

I first met David B. Oliver the way tens of thousands of people have met him—on YouTube. Not everyone would think, "This is a teachable moment" when they hear bad news, but David did and he saw an opportunity and we are better off for it.

David and his wife, Debra Parker Oliver, possessed a deep knowledge gained over their professional lives researching and teaching about aging and end-of-life issues. That he responded to his own deadly illness in a meaningful way is tied both to his character and to his life's work.

David earned a doctorate in sociology and gerontology from the University of Missouri in 1972. He held several academic posts before joining the Heartland Health System where he met and married Debbie. As an administrator, Debbie had helped a small rural hospice acquire Medicare certification. During their life together, she too taught at the university and pursued her interest in applied research to benefit hospice patients. At Heartland, David was responsible for post-acute and chronic care services. He co-authored a book called The Human Factor in Nursing Home Care.

David consistently focused on the importance of engaging in life and living rather than on death and dying. The Olivers produced their first short video shortly after David's diagnosis in the fall of 2011. The diagnosis was Stage 4 nasopharyngeal cancer that begins behind the nose and spreads to lymph nodes and bones.

Scheduled for chemotherapy treatments, David wanted to explain to his medical school colleagues why he would be absent from their upcoming meeting. His condition, he said matter-of-factly, was not curable but it was treatable. Depending on the effectiveness of the treatment, he might live for three to five years or he might live for six months.

A robust man who had run three marathons in the early 1990s, David enjoyed a sprite's sense of humor and a showman's flair for the dramatic, especially as a fan of the football team at the University of Missouri. In the video announcing his illness, he broke out two "puke buckets"—one labeled for college football rivals Kansas Jayhawks and the other for the Oklahoma Sooners. He reassured his colleagues he was going to be all right.

What followed was an outpouring of support and love from colleagues, family, and friends. The video found its way to social media, which widened their circles of support. In the ensuing months, the Olivers produced 28 short videos and an informative e-book called Exit Strategy: Depriving Death of its Strangeness.

On their blog www.dbocancerjourney.blogspot.com, they posted a one-hour presentation to 2,500 attendees at the annual conference of the American Academy of Hospice and Palliative Medicine. Debbie calls that appearance "a professional mountaintop experience" and a "love fest" with an appreciative audience.

Their other videos typically range from three to five minutes each. They offer a remarkable combination of practical advice for those undergoing cancer treatments and for those caring for those who are. They feature David's upbeat, clear, and heartfelt philosophy of living life to its fullest. Most end with a hearty "Go Tigers!" for his beloved Mizzou team. Debbie has her own video, giving the caregiver's perspective. Occasionally their dog Chewy makes an appearance (in one, he can be heard lapping up some water off-camera). The videos' biggest achievement, David believed, was that it made people comfortable about this often-taboo subject.

Debbie did the filming and editing, using a digital camera set on a tripod. They shot mostly in their home although one early video was shot in a salon to immortalize David's hair being shorn prior to chemotherapy. Another was shot at his favorite vacation spot in Loch Vale Lake in Rocky Mountain National Park, Colorado. When it was time, that's where he wanted his ashes scattered.

The quintessential video is the fourth, "The 21 Days In Between," in which David talks about how he feels between rounds of chemotherapy, which he found to have a predictable pattern. He uses a hand-drawn graph to show how days one to four are very good (a green bar); followed by the crash of days five through eight (a long red bar) and nine through 13 (a shorter red bar), followed by the green bar of days 14 to 21, after which there is another round of chemo-therapy.

Consistently ebullient, David is an eloquent spokes-man for the joys of life. He is equally candid about the dark times: his difficult upbringing, his father's alcoholism and suicide, his own struggle with alcohol, his failed first mar-riage. Nor does he mask his fears, his sometime denial about his condition, his frustrations with a health-care system that even he and Debbie—who are as knowledgeable and well-connected as any patients might hope to be—find too often to be brusque, uncoordinated, and insensitive to the ill and to their caregivers. It is the caregivers who suffer most, and who need more support, he emphasizes.

David looks unflinchingly at the impact of illness and the side effects of treatment. He discusses the difficulty of making the decision not to undergo further treatment, and what it will mean to leave the life he loves so much. He talks about what it means to leave his family, his friends, and his colleagues. Though his initial inclination when he was first diagnosed might have been to go to war with the cancer and fight it tooth and nail, he was advised by his 92-year-old men-tor to follow a different path: "One, don't panic; two, don't struggle; three, relax: and four, accept it. It is what it is."

Instead of what David felt would be wasting his time trying to battle the silent killer, he decided that if there ever was a time to teach, this was it.

David went through five months of chemotherapy and unforeseen complications, such as clots in his lungs that caused paralyzing pain one day while he was working at the library. That landed him in the hospital. He retired from his position as a research and teaching professor at the School of Family and Community Medicine at the University of Missouri.

David and Debbie spent the next 15 months traveling, and spending time with their five children and grandchildren. The visited with friends and they made videos. They made decisions about the time David had left.

The cancer returned in June 2013.

By the time I reached out to David and Debbie, I felt I already knew them, having watched their videos and read their book. In real life, they were the same wonderful people I had gotten to know in the digital realm.

That January, David was considering not going for more treatment. He had developed a number of symptoms: fatigue, a deep vein thrombosis, dehydration, continued loss of hearing in one ear. So he thought, let's get certified for hospice care now. But the palliative care team talked them out of it. Let's do another PET scan, they reasoned, to see if the cancer was spreading and, if it was, to devise a palliation strategy, as opposed to "flying in the dark." The Catch-22 of hospice, of course, is that you have to agree to give up any "curative" treatments; even palliative radiation could be interpreted as curative

"I'm a fairly smart guy, but emotionally it was difficult,"

he told me. David was fearful of the results and didn't want the results of the PET scan to change his focus on living.

They talked about doing the next video. He returned to Alcoholics Anonymous to refocus on what is important. Their next video was devoted to how the 12 steps apply to death and dying.

What if David becomes increasingly fatigued, or even bedridden, I asked. Did they plan to continue making videos to share his final decline? Debbie said yes, the plan was to continue although she understood that the burden would fall more on her and she admitted it was already becoming more difficult.

Initially, Debbie had been reluctant to add "video star" to her life as a professional, a wife, mother, grandmother, and now caregiver managing David's care.

"This is my passion and mission, but my natural inclination is to keep my personal life close," she told me. What had swayed her was the realization that working on the videos, the book, and the blog would provide a wider stage and a larger audience than her research ever would. She chose to step up to this opportunity.

In the process, she said, she has had to learn new coping strategies. In the past, her coping strategy was to dive into work. Of her hospice work, she said, "It's more of a ministry than a job. But it meant additional stress."

A good sense of humor helps when caregiving and all it entails gets to be a bit much. She freely admits to sometimes feeling like, if the cancer doesn't kill you, then, I will, she joked. Like David, she believes that caregivers get a lot less attention than they deserve.

"We've got to change that," she said.

David and Debbie were grateful that, with Debbie as caregiver "quarterback," they have had "a continuum of care from diagnosis to our current time," he said, adding: "I'm afraid we're an outlier, a special case."

It's key for the oncology team and the palliative team to coordinate so there's one plan of care, he explained. But generally, "we're not there by a long shot." Continuously, they both stress that we all have to advocate for ourselves.

It felt like a long time between our conversation and Video 25, which was posted in April 2014. It was all about palliative radiation. First we meet Ollie, the Olivers' baby grandson (and half-way into the video, Chewy, the dog, made an appearance, settling on David's lap). By this time, David had been suffering from headaches, vomiting, sore teeth, and extreme fatigue. The fatigue was reduced dramatically after David started using a C-PAP machine. The palliative care doctor believed that apnea had been a cause and that was confirmed in a sleep study. An MRI confirmed that the cancer was back and he chose 20 radiation treatments.

David walks us through the process of being fitted for a mask for his head, which I remembered well from my mother's whole brain radiation treatments. (When she emerged after her first treatment, I joked with her that her face looked like it had been in a waffle iron.) David tells us that the mask made him look and feel like Hannibal Lecter. He admits it took him a while to learn to breathe deeply and relax with the mask affixed to his head. He shows us a graphic of the mask, and a shot of his own waffle-iron face. He named the imposing machine delivering his treatments 'Waldo.'

Video 27 was posted in October 2014. Seated at a picnic table overlooking a crystalline lake at Table Rock State Park in Missouri, David tells us that this may be his last video. "I've been dying to get into hospice," he booms in his customary style, "and guess what? I've finally made it."

"I see my body going," he says, riffing on the idea of his mind and spirit separating from his symptomatic body, which he nicknames "Patch." It's freeing, he says. David is reassuring, as always. Ever the teacher, he explains why he has enrolled in hospice now rather than waiting for the very end stages of illness. He wants to get to know his team and they want to get to know him. He sees his life like a canoe paddling toward a cliff, He assured his hospice team that when the canoe goes over the cliff, they can let him go.

"Life is good," he tells us. "I've had a good ride and I am grateful."

No! was my immediate reaction. In spite of what I know and what I do as a volunteer, I'm still capable of coping by denial. I know I wasn't alone in mourning the eventual loss of a friend.

There was one more video, posted at the end of January 2015. From his familiar chair in the living room, David talks about how, with cancer, there are two patients, not one, stressing, again that the caregiver suffers the most. He acknowledges that he is close to the end, admitting that the hardest thing has been to go from independence to dependence. It's been tough for Debbie, and tough for him, too,

Last Comforts

to hear her weeping at night. He speaks of his deep love for Debbie and of how unimaginably close they've become. Finally, he admonishes, "Doctors, you've got a lot to learn. You've got a lot to accomplish."

David died on March 14, 2015. The announcement came on the blog the next day, saying that "David's Exit Strategy was fulfilled at 7:30 a.m. on March 14—Pi Day. As he had hoped, he died at home, surrounded by others, pain free, and was excited about life until the end."

His two-hour memorial service is posted on the blog. True to form, David makes a final appearance, having taped a short introduction to the service when he was at Table Rock State Park. After leading a Mizzou chant, he says, "The service is going to be great."

I'm grateful for the lessons the Olivers imparted, and for how Magical Elves gave us an intimate glimpse of eight courageous people and their families. What does dying look like? It looks like real life.

Go Tigers!

Chapter 7 Endnote

1. For information about the documentary *Alive Inside*, and about this nonprofit's work in bringing individualized playlists on iPods to people with dementia: https://musicandmemory.org/

8

The Long and Winding Road to Cultural Competence

"Hospice offers the best hope not to be alone, to be with family, to have pain controlled and to be connected to your faith and beliefs. We are as entitled and deserving as anyone else to have these hopes fulfilled."— Richard Payne, MD, Esther Colliflower Professor of Medicine and Divinity at Duke University. [1]

It became apparent to me, as I spent more time as a hospice volunteer, that the overwhelming majority of the people we serve are Caucasian. Are we unique in this way?

Last Comforts

The answer is an emphatic no. While the general population still has a long way to go in becoming better educated about the benefits of palliative and hospice care, the road ahead is even longer for underserved populations, mainly for people of color and for people who are lesbian, gay, bisexual, or transgender (LGBT).

I am a middle-class, heterosexual Caucasian woman, and although I've been able to find common ground with people from a remarkable variety of backgrounds, I know I can't escape the basic lens through which I see the world. It became important to me not only to try to understand other perspectives, but also to learn how some pathfinders are helping the underserved to overcome the hurdles to accessing good care—that remains unseen to so many. I am focusing on the African American and LGBT communities in this chapter because their hurdles have been so high.

African Americans represent fewer than nine percent of the total number of people in hospice care annually, despite representing more than 12 percent of the U.S. population. That figure has remained relatively and stubbornly static since at least 1995, according to the National Hospice and Palliative Care Organization. Behind the statistic is a tangle of cultural and spiritual barriers rooted in our nation's tortured history of racial inequality, discrimination, and violence.

Good care cannot happen without trust between ourselves and those ministering to us. While we have made great progress in seeking to right past injustices, these scars take time, and concerted effort, to heal. The underserved have had more than ample reasons to mistrust our nation's key institutions—chief among them the federal government, law enforcement authorities, and the medical establishment.

Think about the Tuskegee, Alabama, syphilis study for a moment. It began in 1932 and was conducted by the United States Public Health Service on the campus of Tuskegee Institute (the college that Booker T. Washington opened in 1881, now Tuskegee University). The research went on for 40 years—40 years! It was called the "Tuskegee Study of Untreated Syphilis in the Negro Male" and it began with a lie, because researchers never told the more than 600 men enrolled in the study (399 of whom had syphilis; the rest were in a control group) what it was really about. Rather, the men were told that they were to be treated for "bad blood," a commonly used term applied to a variety of ills at the time. The men, most of whom were poor and illiterate sharecroppers, enrolled in the study largely because they were offered free medical care and survivors insurance.

Fifteen years after the study began, penicillin became standard treatment for syphilis. Before that, there were no proven treatments for the disease. And here, the plot thickens. None of the men in the study were treated with penicillin, even after it was recognized as a cure. Not surprisingly, throughout the 40 years of the study, many men died and their wives, children, and others became infected.

But the tide turned after a former Public Health Service investigator contacted an Associated Press reporter who wrote about the experiment. The story ran in New York and Washington in July 1972. Against a backdrop of public outrage, the federal government created an ad hoc panel, with members from the fields of administration, medicine, law, religion, and education to review the study. They concluded that the men had not been given the chance to give informed consent—a basic tenet of health care and research—to the study. They never learned the actual name of the study. They were not told of the consequences of whatever treatments they were to receive, nor about the effect on their wives, girl-friends, and children. They were not given the option to leave the study when it was evident that penicillin could treat and cure the disease. The Tuskegee study ended, officially, one month after the panel issued its report.

Barely a year later, a civil rights attorney filed a class-action suit on behalf of the men in the study and their families. The suit resulted in a settlement giving some $10 million to the study participants. The U.S. government also promised to provide a range of free services—medical and burial—to the survivors and to their wives, widows, and children. The last survivor of that study, a member of the control group, died at 96 of natural causes, in 2004.

No one was prosecuted for what was done to participants.

In May 16, 1997, President Bill Clinton apologized for the Tuskegee study and announced the award of a $200,000 grant to Tuskegee University to initiate plans for a National Center for Bioethics in Research and Health Care. Since then, Tuskegee University received more than $20 million in grants and pledges to help establish and operate the Center, which opened in 1999.

The late Dr. Marian Gray Secundy became the center's

Long Road to Cultural Competence

first director. When it opened, she said, "The entire history of health care in the United States has been shamefully blighted by a long series of racial inequalities. As a result, a legacy of distrust has been handed down from one generation to the next. But this Bioethics Center bears great hope. It takes us to the critical next step in changing the course of history for people of color."

It was fitting, then, that one of the first major steps taken to change that course began with Dr. Secundy and the Bioethics Center. She conceived of what became the first major conference focused on end-of-life care in the African American community. She persuaded the Robert Wood Johnson Foundation (RWJF) to provide the lion's share of its funding (as part of its nationally Targeted End-of-Life Projects Initiative). Before the conference took place, Dr. Secundy relocated from the Bioethics Center to Howard University College of Medicine. After her death, Ethel S. Newman, director of Howard's Program in Health Care Ethics, took responsibility for the RWJF grant. She contracted with Dr. Richard Payne to plan the conference. Payne was then chief of the Pain and Palliative Care Service at Memorial Sloan-Kettering Cancer Center in New York.

The three-day conference drew more than 300 physicians, clergy, educators, policymakers, community leaders, caregivers, medical students, nurses, social workers, and consumer advocates. Featured speakers included Ambassador Andrew Young and the entertainer Della Reese. There were two keynote presentations, 12 workshops, two panel discussions and six plenary sessions. One panel featured six clergy, in recognition of the strong role the church plays in African-American communities, especially regarding the issue of death and dying. In the final session, panelists discussed ways to achieve quality end-of-life care for African Americans.

Following the conference and with an RWJF grant, the Duke Institute on Care at the End of Life produced an e-book featuring 11 commissioned papers on topics related to the most important themes. The entire e-book on End-of-Life Planning for African-Americans, with contributions from some of the leading thinkers who contributed to the groundbreaking conference, is available at:

https://divinity.duke.edu/sites/divinity.duke.edu/files/documents/tmc/KTFULL.pdf

Reading those papers, I was struck, not by how much things have changed since 2004, but how little. Health care disparities persist. African Americans are still less likely than Caucasian Americans to have advance directives. They are more likely to opt for aggressive treatment at the end of life, and are less likely to use hospice care, in part, because they are less informed about it.

Perhaps ironically, then, for nearly a decade, Alabama became a beacon for real progress, where African Americans were accorded the quality care, compassion and dignity that all human beings should have at the end of their lives. The beacon was the Balm of Gilead program at Cooper Green Hospital in Birmingham, where 70 percent of the project's patients were African American.

Balm of Gilead included a 10-bed inpatient facility for those who were dying but had no one to care for them at home. It also provided home-based care for indigent patients, regardless of their ability to pay. One of the more radical things that Balm of Gilead did was to provide comprehensive, team-based care that included doctors, nurses, church groups and volunteers that was integrated into the hospital's acute care system.

Training was a key component. Not only was training instituted for the palliative care staff at the hospital and medical students at the University of Alabama at Birmingham School of Medicine, but it was also provided for church groups, community organizations, and volunteers.

Spearheading the program was F. Amos Bailey, MD, who had completed a fellowship in medical oncology and hematology from 1986 to 1989 at the University of Alabama at Birmingham. After practicing medical oncology for five years in West Virginia, he returned to Birmingham in 1994 as director of the Medical Oncology Clinic at Cooper Green Hospital. Cooper Green was Jefferson County's "safety net" hospital, serving the economically disadvantaged. Bailey also worked in the HIV/AIDS Clinic and became the medical director of the Jefferson County Health Department hospice program.

Now at Denver Health in Colorado, Dr. Bailey told me about his evolution in palliative and hospice care. When approached to be medical director of the hospice program in Birmingham, he recalled, "They said it would be easy," involving signing papers and writing prescriptions, so he agreed.

"I had never done a home visit," he said. "I went to

see a woman at home and it was an epiphany."

They talked and talked—about social supports, emotional issues, the spiritual realm. He was hooked by that experience, he told me, and proceeded to devote a half day each week to home visits. He taught himself about palliative care and read the Oxford Textbook of Palliative Care from cover to cover.

He recognized that at the end of life, the ideal would be for patients to live at home with their families, but for those not in the middle or upper middle class and without those supports, living and dying at home was not a possibility. He persuaded Cooper Green to open an inpatient palliative care program, where patients could be well cared for—cost effectively—in a supportive environment with medical, nursing, social work, and volunteer help.

The key, he said, was that "We weren't going to make people make the terrible choice to give up curative care. We said, 'chemo and antibiotics?' If it's reasonable and could be helpful, we're going to do it. Even ventilators were negotiable.

"And that helped us be successful," he said. "It's what open access hospice is supposed to be about. If you're a poor person and you finally get Medicare, and then someone tries to talk you into giving up treatment [the requirement for hospice care under Medicare rules], it's not fair."

Dr. Bailey and his team applied for an Excellence in End-of-Life Care grant from the Robert Wood Johnson Foundation, whose support enabled Balm of Gilead to open. It was Bailey's strong conviction that Cooper Green would start open-access hospice care whether or not it garnered foundation support.

One reason Balm of Gilead could provide open access hospice, he explained, was that "we had a capitated health-care system." That is, funding—mostly from Medicaid and Medicare, as well as from the county's indigent services fund—provided a set amount of dollars per person, as opposed to a fee-for-service approach. Given that set amount, Cooper Green had the flexibility to decide how best to use precious resources.

After the program was featured [2] on a Bill Moyers PBS series, On Our Own Terms, in 2000, the Birmingham Veterans Administration Medical Center recruited Dr. Bailey to be its Director of Palliative Care. The VA Palliative Care Team has since developed comprehensive programs, including the Safe Harbor Palliative Care Unit, in November 2005. In 2014, Bailey moved to Denver, where he runs an outpatient clinic at the safety net hospital Denver Health 2 ½ days a week for those with serious life-limiting illnesses. He is still involved in a research project for the VA.

The Balm of Gilead program closed at the end of December 2012 when Cooper Green Mercy Hospital closed. Dr. Bailey is justifiably proud of what it achieved, caring for some 500 patients a year. He is white. He was once asked by a visiting African American medical professional how he and his team got patients of color to trust him.

He answered that he approached each patient with this fundamental attitude: "I am here to help you."

His advice to others seeking to reach out to minorities?

Last Comforts

"Your staff needs to be representative of the communities you want to serve, from top to bottom."

A fundamental, yet deeply respectful, approach is also Heidi Barham's calling card. When she meets African American families to counsel them about hospice care, she makes a point of addressing them with the honorific Mr., Ms. or Mrs., and their last names, until she's given permission to use their first names. This practice is consistent with the respect and dignity that etiquette requires but not historically observed. A past chair of the African American Outreach Committee and currently spiritual care coordinator at the Hospice of the Western Reserve in Ohio, Barham is mindful that for so long, African Americans were denied their last names and spoken to, for example, by white employers using only their first names.

The Hospice of the Western Reserve serves northeast Ohio and cares for 1,200 patients on any given day. It holds a free special event every year to reach out to the African-American community, typically attracting several hundred attendees from church groups, social organizations, families, and friends. Its goal is to present facts and dispel common myths about hospice care. At a recent luncheon, a variety of non-profit community organizations provided educational exhibits and free health-care screenings. Attendees were treated to a display of handcrafted art courtesy of the African American Quilt and Doll Guild. The hospice reaches out to the community at health fairs and in churches.

Barham knows that the hospice is making an impact because, of late, people tell her how glad they had been to use the service or how they wish they'd known about hospice sooner. She also finds that clergy are becoming less reticent about helping their congregants facing the end of life. Still, there are misconceptions to dispel, mainly, she told me, that "hospice care is a death sentence; that you've got days or hours left to live." Hospice of the Western Reserve emphasizes the message that the sooner you get involved, the more you benefit. "We're not going to ship you off to a corner," she said. "We're not just going to fill you full of pills. We're not giving up on you."

Barham hears other objections, such as that the ill must have other options, other treatments to pursue. She hears mistrust and resentment, the sense that "You don't want to do anything more for me." She talks about the Tuskegee experiments and about the history of Henrietta Lacks, whose tumor cells were taken unethically by a cell biologist. The taking was unethical in that the scientist did not seek the consent of Mrs. Lacks or that of her family to use her cells to pursue research. In 1951, Mrs. Lacks died of cervical cancer at age 31, four months after giving birth to her fifth child. The cell biologist at Johns Hopkins cut a sliver from her tumor. The cells grew profusely and still grow today, leading to major advances in the development of drugs and vaccines. The family didn't learn that the cells had been taken, or how, until 22 years after her death.

Barham acknowledges that history of an appalling lack of informed consent.

Particularly for a patient suffering from dementia, Barham said it's important to understand "There's a whole history of abuse and mistreatment that comes with that patient. With dementia, the mind is stuck before civil rights and that sets up a fear and mistrust factor."

Mistrust can be triggered by seeing a white male in a white coat. "You do what you can to allay those fears," she said.

It also helps to see people who look like them, she said, an observation that was echoed by Jessica Talley, a social worker, hospice liaison, and market development manager for Hospice of the Chesapeake in Maryland. In 2014, she and Rev. C. Brandon Brewer, that hospice's chaplain-practice manager, put together an education program aimed at health-care providers, social workers, and clergy in Anne Arundel County and Prince George's County. It is titled "Crossing the Jordan: Exploring Ethical and Spiritual Aspects of African-American End-of-Life."

Rev. Brewer said that of the reasons behind the barriers and challenges for minorities in accessing quality end-of-life care, education is most critical. "You can't seek out services if you don't know they exist and are available to you," he told me.

"We want to educate people, not change them," Rev. Brewer noted. Like Hospice of the Western Reserve, they aim to debunk myths about hospice. Most importantly, he said, they emphasize, "You don't have to give up your faith or your culture" if you enter into hospice care.

Talley and Rev. Brewer have made four different formal presentations, typically lasting three hours. So far they've reached about 100 people. Financial resources are limited and they are only two people, so no new presentations were scheduled when I spoke with them. The presentations were well-received, they told me, and clergy in attendance have been eager to take the information back to their congregations.

Language is particularly important in discussing end-of-life issues with African American families, Rev. Brewer and Talley stressed. It makes a big difference to recognize the importance of the spiritual aspect of their lives.

"They don't even like to use the word hospice because it's scary," he said. Instead, they talk about life and living and transitions, as well as the more practical aspects of how the family will be supported, and how they will be cared for at home, if that is where they will be most comfortable."

They also stress that end-of-life care does not interfere with the work of God (or a higher power). "We are not changing God's plan for you," he said.

They recognize that some people feel they must suffer in order to do penance for bad deeds in the past.

"We do not refute a person's beliefs," Rev. Brewer said. "We validate people where they are because it builds a bridge and creates trust. If people say, 'We're praying for a miracle,' my response is, 'I hear you and I join you in that. But if it doesn't happen the way you want it to, what happens then? Let's talk about some other ideas.' "

Talley said that when she tells a family " 'We know God is in control,' their ears are open to me. They relax. They tell me, 'you're speaking my language.' "

Having the right people deliver the messages, with

training and knowledge, is important, she added.

Rev. Brewer said, "Families may come in feeling defeated, but we're about healing. Healing of the soul and mending broken relationships. They matter. Every moment you're alive it matters. Your life has meaning and purpose."

The duo is gratified when people say they have changed their thinking. Rev. Brewer recalled an instance involving a parishioner who is caring for her aging mother. The parishioner had not realized the scope of services available to her, nor did she understand the importance of advance directives. She requested an advance directive package to bring to her family. Nurses and social workers have commented that they had no ideas of the complexities or the barriers involved, Talley said. Hearing about the fears of nurses and social workers of not sufficiently understanding the cultural issues fascinates her.

The spirituality component was new for many health-care workers, too.

I asked, "If you had a magic wand, how would you change things? What would you like to see happen?"

Rev. Brewer's reply: "The blinders would be removed and people would see hospice for what it is. There would be equal participation. We want to see African Americans have the same peaceful life closure as other groups."

Going Back Into the Closet

Earl Collom is a social worker and liaison in Manhattan for the Visiting Nurse Service of New York Hospice and

Long Road to Cultural Competence

Palliative Care. Once, he visited one gay client and noticed many photos of people, places, friends, and travel displayed on the apartment's walls and shelves. During his next visit, many had been removed. When Collom asked why, the client replied, "I didn't want to offend anyone."

Imagine yourself living at home—frail, ill and experiencing the most vulnerable time of your life. Imagine being worried that whoever is assigned to assist you is hostile to the way you've lived your life. What would you do? Would you hide who you are? Would you refer to your partner or spouse as a roommate? Sadly, for elders who are gay, lesbian, bisexual, or transgender and contending with advanced illness, going back into the closet out of fear of neglect, disapproval, or abuse is not uncommon.

Their fear is based on reality. Until recently, homosexuality was considered a mental disorder, and still is thought of as a moral failing among some segments of the population. A gay man or a lesbian could be jailed or sent to a mental institution. For much of the 20th century, this country's major institutions—government, the military, and police— perpetrated the bias. In the 1950s, the American Psychiatric Association identified homosexuality as a mental disorder. In the 1970s, the U.S. Supreme Court refused to hear the case of a teacher fired for lesbianism, thus making it legal to fire teachers for being LGBT. For more examples of the sorry history of bias and discrimination, see www.forge-forward.ort/tan.

The National Resource Center on LGBT Aging has found that LGBT elders are five times less likely to seek health and human services than heterosexuals because of fear of harassment and discrimination. About a quarter of transgender people report being denied equal health care (or refused outright) with Latino transgender people reporting the highest rate of unequal treatment.

For LGBT elders, end-of-life care may not follow the model of having caregiver support provided by family members. More likely to live alone, they are less likely to have children care for them than their heterosexual peers. According to a 2011 national health study co-authored by the Center for American Progress and also by Services and Advocacy for Gay, Lesbian, Bisexual, and Transgender Elders (SAGE), social isolation remains a major issue as LGBT seniors are three to four times less likely to have children, twice as likely to live alone, and twice as likely to be single.

Moreover, they may be in poorer financial straits than their heterosexual peers with the result that the need for care is acute. The resource center estimated that in 2010 there were between 1.6 and 2.4 million gay and lesbian elders in the U.S. and that by 2030 there will be as many as 7 million.

In Spring 2011, six organizations that advocate for elders and for the LGBT population published "LGBT Older Adults in Long-Term Care Facilities: Stories from the Field." [3]

The study was conducted between October 2009 and June 2010 in 44 states and the District of Columbia. It includes 769 individuals who identified themselves as LGBT seniors. In some cases, their family members, friends, and social service providers identified them. Among the highlights:

Did these older adults feel that they could be open about their sexual orientation with staff at a nursing home, assisted living, or other long-term care facility?

Only 22 percent replied "yes."

What did they expect would be the consequences if they did come out in such a setting? In order of priority, they identified discrimination by staff; discrimination by other residents; isolation from other residents; abuse or neglect by staff.

Of those who lived in long-term facilities, or cared for those who did, the most frequently reported problem was negative treatment from other residents, followed by verbal or physical harassment by staff. Moreover, 51 percent reported staff refusing to provide basic care (such as toileting, bathing, or feeding).

Reading the statistics can be upsetting. But reading the comments of some of the people who responded to the study is heartbreaking. A litany of sorrows and stories of lives derailed, couples separated by family members who had legal authority over the facility resident; feelings of loneliness and isolation because of disapproval by other residents or staff; having aides attempting to get people to "repent" for their sins; choosing to go back into the closet for fear of neglect or harm. A link to the study: http://www.nsclc.org/wp-content/uploads/2011/07/LGBT-Stories-from-the-Field.pdf [4]

Powerful, too, are the stories of the people we come to know in filmmaker Stu Maddux's 2011 documentary, *Gen Silent*, which documents the experience of six LGBT elders in the Boston area. We meet Lawrence Johnson and Alexandre Rheume, a couple who had been together for 38 years until Rheume's Parkinson's disease compelled them to seek professional care for him. At first, Rheume moved to an assisted living development, but they both felt unwanted, uncomfortable, and judged, when Johnson did simple things, such as feeding or holding his partner's hand. Rheume moved to a nursing home that felt more welcoming. But caregiving and grief took its toll on Johnson, who became increasingly isolated, depressed, and suicidal. He began to write poetry and gradually began a new chapter in his own life.

We meet Sheri Barden and Lois Johnson, a married lesbian couple who have long been advocates for LGBT rights. In the course of learning their story, we hear about how a Boston newspaper in the 1950s made it a practice of outing people, and how people took to using fake names as one tactic to avoid being identified. We learn how the FBI tailed people after rallies in the 1960s. Now Barden and Johnson are hoping to be able to age in place, but if illness forced one or both to have to move, Johnson said she might hide the nature of their relationship; Barden would not.

We also meet KrisAnne Hembrough, a transgender woman struggling with terminal illness. A Vietnam War veteran, she became a woman in 2003. She feared how she would be treated in the healthcare system. Indeed, when a crisis prompts an emergency trip to the hospital, it is the filmmaker who the emergency medical technician contacts to learn whether KrisAnne is fully transgender. Long estranged from her family, KrisAnne does reconnect briefly with her grown son. In her final days, a group of volunteers, cobbled together by a social worker, provide her with companionship and validation.

Long Road to Cultural Competence

The documentary features activists such as Bob Linscott, who spearheads Café Emmanuel, a community meal program specifically for LGBT elders and their friends. So many live alone and are estranged from their families, he said, that when the organization asked people to fill out a form listing their emergency contacts, some did not know of anyone to name.

The Café itself became a support network.

What drew the filmmaker Maddux, a man in his '40s, to these stories of elders? My mother would have called him an old soul, but beyond that, he told me that as a gay man, he felt he had a distinct lack of role models in his life and wanted to investigate the reasons why.

The answer: they're invisible. Scared to be out. "So it was personal for me," he said. He worked with Boston's LGBT Aging Project, which found likely subjects, and worked on the film for two years, including six months in pre-production; following and filming his subjects for a year; and another six months in post-production.

The film has been shown hundreds of times not only at film festivals but also at health-care conferences, government agencies, colleges and universities, houses of worship, Fortune 500 companies, and aging services organizations. It has become a training tool for some, a fundraising tool for others.

"I'm always taken aback by the number of people who don't think LGBT and elders in the same sentence," he said. "There's no media representation. They're invisible as a group."

Last Comforts

It may well be true that baby boomers will not follow in their elders' footsteps by returning to the closet when they need health-care services.

In the meantime, what can be done for the elder LGBT population?

As Dale Mitchell, an LGBT advocate in Boston, remarked in *Gen Silent*, the amount of training currently underway for aging services and health-care organizations is like "a gnat on the side of an elephant." But there are exceptions.

I met Tim Johnston, PhD, manager of education and training for the National Resource Center on LGBT Aging, a federally funded project of SAGE (the Center for American Progress and Services and Advocacy for Gay, Lesbian, Bisexual, and Transgender Elders). We met following his presentation on creating safe and inclusive services for LGBT older adults at Barnabas Health Hospice and Palliative Care Center's annual "Living to the End" conference in fall 2014.

He presented a shortened version of the several-hours' long training he typically gives. He addressed nurses, aides, and social workers in attendance with a taste of the basics. That included definitions, case studies of several LGBT individuals representing common issues that arise, the unique challenges of transgender people, a brief history of the highlights (or lowlights) of major developments in the 20th and 21st century, and ways to begin creating LGBT-inclusive services.

He stressed that many health care, social services, and long-term care facilities assume that they simply do not have any LGBT clients. Assume that you do, he said. Don't wait

Long Road to Cultural Competence

for self-disclosure and make it clear that all families—biological and families of choice—are welcome. Among other recommendations: Ask clients about their sexual and gender identity in a safe and confidential manner. Ask open-ended questions, such as, who do you consider family? Or, who in your life is especially important? Staff should know and use the correct pronoun that their clients prefer. Respect gender identity when providing sex-segregated services. Promote diversity and inclusion within your organization. Promote cultural competency training.

One large organization that has been committed to cultural competency training is the 97-year-old, 870-bed Hebrew Home of Riverdale in New York City. COO David Pomeranz told me that for two years, everyone from executives—including Pomeranz—down to line staff has been taking part in SAGE training. Some changes involve an assessment of marketing materials, activities, and events, which had been skewed heterosexual.

With a highly diverse staff of 2,000, staff response to the training has varied; some are resistant while others are glad to participate and wish it had happened sooner. Pomeranz estimated it will take five years for everyone to "get it," he said.

Hebrew Home has not had any transgender residents yet, Pomeranz told me. What is new is a social daycare program with SAGE. It is believed to be the first inclusive social adult day program for LGBT seniors in New York State.

SAGE and VNSNY teamed up to provide training to VNSNY's extensive health care employees and clinicians.

Last Comforts

Earl Collom made the connection between the organizations. At an initial meeting in April 2012 with senior leadership of both groups, Collom realized that "The big assumption—that clinicians knew about LGBT people and understood their needs—was wrong. In health care, there's an element of negativity, bias, prejudice, mistreatment at times."

It is important to educate staff. Collom said, "Unless you understand the baggage of someone 65-plus, you can't provide holistic treatment. They are not comfortable disclosing orientation. They are always monitoring the safety of [a particular] setting because of that historic baggage."

Discrimination based on sexual preference or gender identity may be against the law, but as Collom remarked, "Statutory changes in regulations don't necessarily translate into personal beliefs. Healthcare professionals in New York come from lots of places, including some where they have no non-discrimination laws."

The next step was to propose to VNSNY a curriculum that would be taught to hospice clinicians and would be mandatory in-service training for all new employees. When I met Collom, he told me that training was underway in the city's boroughs. He wanted to extend the training to the rest of VNSNY, not just the hospice and palliative care staff. He also wanted to see the training regarding bisexual and transgender elders evolve too, as those issues are more complex than gay and lesbian issues. During training, he's had hospice social workers ask, 'Can I legally ask those questions' [about sexual orientation, gender identity and expression, lifestyle] or, 'Why do I need to ask those questions?' That tells him they are not comfortable with it and don't necessarily know what to do with the answer.

"That's the change event—when we train our clinicians to ask the question," he said.

Collom himself has been doing hospice work for more than nine years and is more than comfortable asking the question. It can be a matter of asking who the person lives with, or whose name is on an apartment lease.

"It should be a nothing question, like asking if they're a veteran," he said. "My perspective is to establish a safe zone at the beginning of any meetings with our residents, to help them wrap up, and resolve issues. There are so many loose ends: family estrangement, families of choice, what residual hurts remain?"

What he finds rewarding is providing quality care in the last phases of someone's life. He's done that for a long time. His career dates back to the AIDS crisis, including 10 years as admissions director of Rivington House, New York City's only LGBT-oriented nursing home that catered to AIDS patients. It closed in 2014.

Collom was married a year when we met though he's been with his husband for 22 years. He is optimistic that LGBT baby boomers will approach end-of-life care without the baggage that plagues their elders. "They have a voice and will use it."

Collom is optimistic that in time there will be more acceptance and less bias against the LGBT population. What seemed so telling to me is that in the meantime—in the heart of what is arguably one of the most progressive cities in the nation—Collom himself admitted to having second thoughts, should he ever have to enter a nursing home for care.

In early 2015, SAGE opened an LGBT-friendly senior community center in the Bronx, which is open five days a week and serves hot meals. It also offers yoga and tai chi lessons, a media room, bilingual English-Spanish programs, and a reading club. (SAGE already had centers in midtown Manhattan, Staten Island, Harlem, and Brooklyn.) The Bronx center has $1.5 million in city funding. An elder gay man explained to a New York Times reporter that for some time he had been taking the long subway ride to the SAGE senior center in midtown Manhattan, rather than go to senior centers in the Bronx where he never felt welcome.

"I think we need our own places," he said.

Is that the answer? For those dealing with serious illness, are LGBT-focused assisted living, continuing-care communities, or nursing homes the answer?

I asked filmmaker Greg Maddux how he felt about that.

"The older I get, the more I want to be with people like me," he said. "I would like an environment that's not just welcoming but celebratory."

In fact, there are a handful of such communities. Some, like Triangle Square and Argyle apartment buildings in Hollywood, and the John C. Anderson apartments in Philadelphia, are affordable rentals while others, like Fountaingrove Lodge continuing care development in Santa Rosa, California are quite pricey.

Oakmont Senior Living, a private developer that owns

Long Road to Cultural Competence

and manages about a dozen senior living facilities in California, built the $52 million, LGBT-focused Fountaingrove Lodge on 10 acres overlooking a golf course. It features 64 independent living apartments, six standalone bungalows, and a 27-unit memory-care wing. Designed in Craftsman style, it has a fitness and wellness center, a pool, 22-seat theater, wine cellar, bistro, and second floor dining room, plus a concierge, activities director, and transportation service. The apartments are comfortably sized from over 800 to about 2,000 square feet. Residing there does not come cheap. When it opened in 2013, entry fees started at just under $200,000 and rose to over $900,000, while monthly fees started at over $3,000.

Michael Dively moved to Fountaingrove Lodge in May 2014 at age 76 and shared the story of his personal odyssey with me. At 43, he'd come out as gay, moved to Key West to explore his sexuality, and lived there for 20 years. More recently, he decided he did not want to live the rest of his days in Key West. Health care was "mediocre," he said, and there were no assisted-living residences there. While exploring options, he lived for five years in Santa Cruz, California and assumed that when he turned 80, he would likely move to an independent living development.

Dively clearly values community. A philanthropist, he lived happily in Santa Cruz, and had developed close ties there in the Quaker community as well as with gay youth organizations (through his foundation, the Mukti Fund). He taught, and swam competitively. He told me the one assisted-living development in Santa Cruz did not seem to have any gay or lesbian residents—or if they were there, they were closeted.

Last Comforts

A close friend of his from Key West learned of Fountaingrove Lodge and, following its groundbreaking, both signed on to its mailing list. When the friend's partner died, he started thinking seriously about moving. But Dively, being healthy and actively engaged in his Santa Cruz community, had doubts about moving to a continuing-care development. He consulted with a Quaker friend who advises elders about housing options. She convinced him that people often move too late and, for him, it was the ideal time to become involved with Santa Rosa and his prospective neighbors. Dively and his Key West friend decided: "If you do it, I'll do it."

Separately, they moved into Fountaingrove Lodge in May 2014.

Dively has become involved here, too. He chairs the wellness committee and meditates regularly with a half-dozen residents. He co-chairs Caring Community, a group that explores the idea of how they, as volunteers, can provide care to other residents.

"I like the energy here," he said, extolling the development design, his fairway views, the morning sun in his apartment, and the oak trees in the backyard. As the development is not fully occupied, he noted that the developers are now marketing more broadly, beyond San Francisco, to Los Angeles, Miami, Chicago, and New York. His neighbors are mostly in their sixties and seventies, although one resident is 89—"a role model for me," he said. A few of his neighbors are heterosexual. One couple has three grown children, two of whom are gay; they wanted a place where their children could feel comfortable visiting, as does a woman whose grandchild is gay.

Is Fountaingrove Lodge a golden ghetto? Will there no longer be a need for developments like this by the time the baby boomers need it?

Dively said, "That's my fantasy—that things will continue to get better."

He likened his hope to the Woman's Club of Key West, a service organization begun in the 1890s. Its membership had been open only to women. In the late 1990s, the club began accepting men as members as there was no longer a need for a club where only women could be members.

"In the decades ahead it will be easier to come out, to get jobs, and in retirement years, to be accepted," he said. Right now, he added, it's unfair and scary to think that you could be in the most vulnerable state and be treated by a nurse holding a Bible while condemning your sexual orientation.

By contrast, Fountaingrove Lodge is a safe environment, where residents can feel comfortable and not have to explain or defend themselves. That is important. As Earl Collom, the New York social worker, said, "You should have only one death in your life, without having people killing your past."

Chapter 8 Endnotes

1. Dr. Richard Payne was the founder of the Initiative to Improve Palliative Care for African Americans, a project of Open Society Institute's Project on Death in America (1994–2003). Payne is director of the Institute on Care at the End of Life at the Divinity School at Duke University in Durham, NC. The e-book on *End-of-Life Planning for African-Americans,* with contributions from Dr. Payne and other leading thinkers who contributed to the "Last Miles of the Way Home" conference in 2004, is available at: https://divinity.duke.edu/sites/divinity.duke.edu/files/documents/tmc/KTFULL.pdf www.tuskegee.edu/about_us/centers_of_excellence/bioethics_center/about_the_center.aspx

2. On Our Own Terms. www.pbs.org/wnet/onourownterms/about/

3. www.nsclc.org/wp-content/uploads/2011/07/LGBT-Stories-from-the-Field.pdf

The study is also accessible at www.justiceinaging.org. While there, see also "20 Common Nursing Home Problems—And How to Resolve Them," a useful document for all. Another helpful resource is "Creating End-of-Life Documents for Trans Individuals" by Corey Prachniak, Esq., at the National Resource Center on LGBT Aging: www.lgbtagingcenter.org.

9

Educating Physicians: Learning How to Talk the Talk

66 I was required to prove my competence with inserting central line catheters, leading Code Blues, performing lumbar punctures, drawing blood, and obtaining arterial blood-gas samples. But not a single senior physician needed to certify that I could actually speak to patients about medical care." —Dr. Angelo Volandes, on the process of his becoming a board-certified physician during his residency at

the University of Pennsylvania. He is the author of *The Conversation: A Revolutionary Plan for End-of-Life Care.* [1]

Once, out of curiosity, I asked my primary care physician—who is considerably younger than I am—what kind of training she'd had in end-of-life issues. Her response was, "None." (To be fair, she did tell me the hospital where she is affiliated requires its physicians to take a course in pain management.) I do have an advance directive tucked away somewhere in her office files, though we've never discussed it.

I began to wonder: What do physicians in training need to know about advanced illness and the end of life? How do they learn about how to talk with patients and families, particularly if they have bad news to impart? When do they learn how to work with an interdisciplinary team to give their patients their best possible quality of life? Do they see what dying looks like, as they say, up close and personal?

The fact is, medical education requirements are simply not uniform. While medical schools require curriculum coverage of end-of-life care, the average total offering is only 17 hours over the 4 years. The Institute of Medicine's Dying in America report notes that medical schools don't usually require a course to address this topic. [2]

In 2000 the Liaison Committee for Medical Education (LCME), which accredits medical education programs leading to the MD degree in the U.S. and Canada, began requiring that accredited U.S. medical schools teach end-of-life care, but it does not provide guidelines for precisely how to do that. In LCME's most current standards for accreditation, the words "palliative" and "hospice" do not appear at all; its one and only reference to end-of-life appears in its standards concerning organ systems. [3]

It is not surprising that a 2008 study in the Journal of Palliative Medicine reported that of 128 U.S. medical schools queried, palliative and hospice care was a required course in less than 16 percent of the 47 that responded, and a required rotation in only 19 percent. [4] Fifteen percent offered an elective course and 29 percent an elective rotation. The study pointed to the lack of established guidelines to define what palliative care training should cover; and to the lack of mandated objectives and competencies on which to base on an audit of a medical school's curriculum.

In the absence of guidelines, one educational standout is Albany Medical College in New York State, where beginning in 2006, third-year medical students have been required to do a one-week hospice rotation. The rotations are done in collaboration with Community Hospice, which serves the seriously ill in eight counties in upstate New York. Following the rotation, the students write an essay about the three most important things they have learned from their experiences.

Dr. John A. Balint is the chief architect of the hospice rotation. He has been with Albany Medical College for more than 50 years, starting as head of the Division of Gastroenterology, then chair of the Department of Medicine in 1981. He developed the Center for Medical Ethics Education and Research (now the Alden March Bioethics Institute) in 1994.

The program is "one of my joys in this world," Dr. Balint told me. It began with a conversation he had with the medical school director at a time when the school was undergoing a major retooling of its curriculum. Dr. Balint, who had served on a hospice board for eight years, decided that adding the hospice rotation would be an important complement to the bioethics program.

"This exposure makes a huge difference," he said. " 'There's nothing more I can offer you;' our students don't say that anymore. Rather, they learn to say 'I can give you a transition to another kind of life and I'll be with you throughout.' "

He added: "Students get a sense of what it's like to be a patient. They hear stories of so many varieties."

He told me about how one student learned that he shared a birthday with one of the patients; how touched and amazed he was that, despite being close to death, the patient was keenly interested in the student's education and his hopes and plans.

"It is remarkable to learn that kind of thing," he said.

An article about medical students' perspectives on the impact of this hospice rotation appeared in the Journal of Palliative Medicine in 2011. [5] It chronicled the experience of 104 third-year students who had completed their rotation and written essays about their experience during the academic year of 2006–7.

Of the many themes that echoed throughout the essays, the most prominent was how the students came to understand the benefits and philosophy of hospice. Chief among them was learning the practice of caring for the whole person; the idea of non-abandonment; and understanding that death is a natural part of life and not a sign of failure.

Educating Physicians to Talk the Talk

"Hospice [care] is a success when, during patients' final moments, one can celebrate the beauty of life rather than the sorrow of death," one student wrote.

Moreover, students said that their experience gave them a better understanding of how to talk to future patients about hospice care. The skills they learned—particularly the importance of being present and willing to listen to patients—would transfer to any patient care setting.

The students also came to understand the value of working with an interdisciplinary team and to appreciate the skills of different team members in addressing the many different kinds of suffering they encountered.

"I learned about the scope of suffering—the many ways a person can suffer—beyond the scope of physical suffering," one student wrote. Another said, "Comfort care involves the same high level of clinical reasoning... as curative care."

Still another student wrote, "Some of the best medicine does not consist of medications at all."

Many students were deeply moved by their connections with patients. One student wrote, "Bearing witness to someone's long, full life or the tragedy surrounding their too-soon death was a remarkable thing to feel part of."

Dr. Balint said, "We are hoping to do a follow-up study to ask students after residency how much of what they learned improved how they practice."

Medical school curricula vary widely. In addition to standard classroom teaching and small group work, some require students to engage in role play with actors playing

Last Comforts

different scenarios to hone their communication skills. Some schools include education about advance care planning and goals of care. At Robert Wood Johnson Medical School in New Jersey, the curriculum requires students to take classes in patient-centered care from their first year through the end of their fourth year.

James C. Salwitz, MD is a medical oncologist, a clinical professor at Rutgers' Robert Wood Johnson Medical School, and a prolific blogger. He frequently lectures both at the school and in the community on topics related to cancer care, hospice, and palliative medicine.

Dr. Salwitz believes that death is not the enemy but that suffering is. He explained that as a medical oncologist, he's aware that eventually his patients will die and that understanding the cycle of life is critical to avoiding burnout as a physician.

"So you always have to have something to offer your patients," he said. "I tell students that this is part of your job. You have to be able to answer really tough questions. Your job is to help [patients] live. Just being at the bedside is infinitely powerful."

He began teaching about death and dying in 1989 and finds his students in the second, third, and fourth years very open to the subject.

"They still have the basic desire to help," he said. "They go through emotions and experiences they don't get anywhere else in life. They become aware of their own mortality. This helps them cope with that, and with what their relationships with patients will be in the future."

Educating Physicians to Talk the Talk

The Growth of Palliative Care

Beyond medical school, education in palliative care is growing at the resident and fellowship level. The American Board of Internal Medicine, which certifies internists, now requires residency training to incorporate care of the dying. It has developed a guide to define physician competence in end-of-life care for residency programs. In June 2006, the Accreditation Council for Graduate Medical Education began the process of accreditation for hospice and palliative medicine fellowship programs.

Looking at residency education, the Institute of Medicine Committee on Approaching Death notes that "Residency programs will have to place more emphasis on these issues and provide training opportunities in hospices and home care settings."

According to the American Academy of Hospice and Palliative Medicine (AAHPM), 107 palliative care fellowships are scheduled for the 2016–17 academic year. Certification programs in palliative care were established for seven levels of nursing, two levels of social work, and chaplaincy.

Palliative care is a relatively young specialty. In September 2006, the American Board of Medical Specialties approved the creation of hospice and palliative medicine as a subspecialty of 10 participating boards. In 2015, more than 6,500 physicians are board-certified in palliative care, according to the AAHPM.

The number of U.S. hospitals offering palliative care services is increasing too. Annual surveys by the American

Last Comforts

Hospital Association, along with data from the National Palliative Care Registry, reports that in U.S. hospitals with 50 or more beds, palliative care programs increased from 658 in 2000 to more than 1,700 in 2012, [6] 61 percent of all hospitals that size.

(The 248-bed community hospital where my father spent his last months now offers palliative care services.)

The Joint Commission is the independent accreditation and certification agency for the more than 20,500 health care organizations and programs in the United States. In 2011, the Joint Commission initiated an advanced certification program for palliative care. The certification recognizes hospital inpatient programs that demonstrate exceptional patient and family-centered care that optimizes the quality of life for patients with serious illnesses.

David Casarett, MD, expects palliative medicine to grow in size and importance over the next five to ten years, with greater integration into all facets of health care. Casarett is the chief medical officer for hospice and palliative care at the University of Pennsylvania Perelman School of Medicine. He foresees more funding, either through public or foundation support, to provide palliative care outside the hospital setting.

One obstacle is that "palliative care is still a money loser," Casarett said. "You can't bill as much as a cardiologist, or bring in as much revenue. There has to be recognition that what we do has value."

The supply of palliative and hospice care specialists does not meet the present need. If current trends continue,

Educating Physicians to Talk the Talk

the shortage is likely to continue in the next decade and beyond. Palliative care advocates foresee an increasing need for such care to be available not just in hospitals but also in the community and in the home, an idea that has been slow to achieve traction due in part to the limited number of specialists available.

Spurred by anecdotal evidence, in 2008, the American Academy of Hospice and Palliative Medicine appointed a task force to assess whether a palliative care physician shortage existed, and to determine the optimal number of such physicians. In a December 2010 article [7] in the Journal of Pain and Symptom Management, Dale Lupu summarized the task force conclusion affirming an acute shortage of palliative care physicians while noting that the capacity of fellowship programs to fill the shortage was insufficient.

"Either we retrain existing physicians in the skills of hospice and palliative medicine or we bring new physicians into this practice capacity... An educational pathway that invites interested, experienced physicians to engage in additional training is... one solution to the shortage," Lupu wrote.

AAHPM joins the prestigious Institute of Medicine in advocating for a "palliative training for all" approach. In its Dying in America report, the IOM noted: "The number of hospice and palliative care specialists is small, which means the need for palliative care also must be met through primary care and through the other clinical specialties that entail care for significant numbers of people nearing the end of life (for example, cardiology, oncology, pulmonology, and nephrology)."

155

Last Comforts

The Institute of Medicine recommended: "All clinicians across disciplines and specialties who care for people with advanced serious illness should be competent in basic palliative care, including communication skills, interprofessional collaboration and symptom management."

The IOM decried the "persistence of single-profession education silos," which is problematic because palliative care relies on a team-based approach.

Critical, too, in the IOM view, is that while "studies have established that physicians can be taught the communication skills needed to provide good end-of-life care, few medical educators teach these skills."

Among the IOM's major recommendations is that "educational institutions, credentialing bodies, accrediting boards, state regulatory agencies, and health care delivery organizations should establish the appropriate training, certification, and/or licensure requirements to strengthen the palliative care knowledge and skills of all clinicians who care for individuals with advanced serious illness who are nearing the end of life."

IOM recommends that educational institutions and professional societies provide training in palliative care throughout each professional's career. To do so, these organizations should "commit institutional resources to increasing the number of available training positions for specialty-level palliative care."

In the meantime, some institutions are beefing up their training in physician communication skills. At Memorial Sloan Kettering Cancer Center in New York City, the goals

Educating Physicians to Talk the Talk

of the communication skills research and training program are to help surgeons, oncologists, and others to communicate better. The dedicated staff of trainers works in laboratory space that includes a classroom and six video-recording training rooms. Attending physicians, fellows, and residents from Sloan Kettering and other institutions take part in the training.

The curriculum includes modules covering breaking bad news; shared decision-making about treatment options; responding to patient anger; communicating with patients via interpreters; discussing prognosis; discussing transition from curative to palliative care; death, dying and end-of-life goals of care; and conducting a family meeting.

In Harrisburg, Pennsylvania, Pinnacle Health System developed a physician-training program to improve doctors' communication with their patients after a baseline assessment showed they needed to improve. For example, physicians introduced themselves to patients only about one quarter of the time; brief conversations were common; and a lack of empathy was evident. Since then, the training program has helped 250 physicians improve their skills and probably not coincidentally, patient satisfaction climbed dramatically.

"We need to move away from the perception that social skills and better communication are a kind of optional extra for doctors," Nirmal Joshi, chief medical officer of Pinnacle Health System, wrote in January 2015 in an op-ed in *The New York Times*. "A good bedside manner is simply good medicine."

Last Comforts

Addressing deficits in physicians' communication skills is not new. In 1992, the late Dr. Robert Buckman wrote about how health-care professionals break bad news [8] to patients and their families. In 1998, he and Dr. Walter Baile of the MD Anderson Cancer Canter presented their six-step communications guide to the American Society of Clinical Oncologists.

I am summarizing those steps here because they seem to me to be a Platonic ideal of how meetings should take place among people who are seriously ill, their caregivers, and the physicians charged with their care. The first letter of each step begins with a letter in the acronym SPIKES, which is the name of the communications guide.

1. S—Setting up the Interview. Buckman and Baile advise clinicians to mentally rehearse a patient meeting and to anticipate emotional reactions and tough questions, bearing in mind how important it is for the patient to get the information to enable planning for the future. A private setting, such as a conference room, is ideal and it should include caregivers. The clinician should sit, to indicate the meeting will not be rushed. Buckman and Baile recommend maintaining eye contact to establish rapport and, if the patient is comfortable with this, touching the patient on the arm or holding a hand.

2. P—Assessing the Patient's Perception. "Before you tell, ask." That means the clinician should learn what the patient's understanding is of his or her medical situation. That gives the clinician a chance to correct misinformation and to frame the bad news in the context of what the patient understands.

Educating Physicians to Talk the Talk

3: I—Obtaining the Patient's Invitation. Sometimes patients don't want full information. At this point, a physician might ask, "How would you like me to give the information about [scheduled] test results? Would you like me to give you all the information or sketch out the results and spend more time discussing the treatment plan?" The physician can also offer to answer any of the patient's questions in the future, or offer to talk to a relative or friend.

4: K—Giving Knowledge and Information to the Patient. A heads-up that bad news is in the offing may lessen the blow of the actual news. On the other hand, excessive bluntness should be avoided (as in, "You have very bad cancer and unless you get treatment immediately you are going to die.") Useful phrases could be: "Unfortunately I've got some bad news to tell you" or "I'm sorry to tell you that…"

Physicians should try to avoid medical and technical jargon and should keep checking to determine the patient's level of understanding. Even if the prognosis is poor, physicians should not use phrases like "there is nothing more we can do for you."

STEP 5: E—Addressing the Patient's Emotions with Empathic Responses. It's a shock to hear bad news and understandably, on hearing bad news, patients can react emotionally, including crying, anger, denial, or disbelief. This is a time for the physician to offer support and solidarity with an empathic response. That means observing the patient's emotion; asking open questions about how the patient is thinking or feeling; identifying the reason for the emotion; and making a "connecting statement" acknowledging the patient's feelings.

STEP 6: S—Strategy and Summary. This is the "where do we go from here" step. The patient's wishes and goals are an important part of decision-making. Physicians should ask if the patient is ready to discuss a treatment plan.

A small cottage industry is evolving from Buckman and Baile's recommendations. They use online learning, videos, social media, and apps along with in-person, continuing education, and "train the trainer" courses. VitalTalk, for example, a nonprofit, teaches that physician communication skills can be learned, with practice, a map, and with feedback. VitalTalk is based on the insights of its founders, Dr. Anthony Back, professor of medicine at both the University of Washington and the Fred Hutchinson Cancer Research Center, and colleagues Robert M. Arnold, MD; Kelly Edwards, PhD; and James Tulsky, MD.

The VitalTalk website features videos and eight, one-page guides (which they call "talking maps") that cover a range of topics, from talking about dying, to transitions in goals of care, managing conflicts, respecting and responding to patients' emotions and more. The guides are simple, clear-cut, and eminently sensible. They're worth a look by either a patient or caregiver because each of us would want our physicians to communicate with us with the kind of clarity and empathy these guides espouse. [9]

As Dr. Back explains in an introductory video, good communication is not just about being more "empathic." It is in service to what the physician needs to do; it's about people.

Educating Physicians to Talk the Talk

As physicians become better communicators, he believes, they will see themselves more as a guide than a fixer—a "richer place to be," he says.

The VitalTalk app provides a five-step GUIDE (an acronym for Get Ready; Understand; Inform; Deepen; and Equip) to giving serious or bad news. Physicians can also access instructive videos and offer users a "debriefing" feature to review notes from patient meetings.

Dr. Angelo Volandes, who practices internal medicine at Massachusetts General Hospital, co-founded Advance Care Planning Decisions, a non-profit foundation where the mission is to empower patients and their families with video tools to support decision-making.

In his book *The Conversation: A Revolutionary Plan for End-of-Life Care*, Dr. Volandes acknowledges that "If the ten years of my undergraduate and graduate medical education were plotted onto a single calendar year, the amount of time I spent learning to talk with patients about medical care would likely last a single day. The other 364 are spent learning about everything else in medicine."

Dr. Volandes wanted to help his patients make informed choices about their care. In his book, he tells the story of taking a patient with a brain tumor and her husband on a tour of the hospital ICU, to give them a sense of what different kinds of measures, such as CPR, ventilation, and intubation are about. Inadvertently, they witnessed a Code Blue, with doctors and nurses feverishly administering CPR on an elderly man. The next day, the patient made up her mind not to opt for life-prolonging measures. She went home with hospice care. He took other patients and their families on ICU tours, too, mostly at night when it was quiet, and discussed the "messy, clinical details" involved in various diseases. The ICU nurses called a halt to the tours.

He began to think, what about an educational video? He devoted a year to research, which involved interviewing many seriously ill people and their families for their views about decision-making. He met with medical specialists, nurses, social workers, and chaplains. Among other insights, he learned that patients' choices fell into three general categories: (life-prolonging) full code; comfort care; and a middle approach consisting of limited medical care. The following year, Dr. Volandes and his research group got permission from patients to film them at home, in the ICU, in nursing homes, and in a dialysis unit.

One striking thing about how the videos were developed: Dr. Volandes and his team—including his wife, Dr. Althea Delight Davis—took special care to make sure the videos would be as unbiased as possible. They would not advocate for any one approach, such as "do everything," "do nothing," or "provide limited care." Experts in medicine, geriatrics, oncology, cardiology, ethics, and decision-making reviewed the videos. Also striking, is evidence that shows that people who learn about end-of-life choices through video, compared with those who learn about their options verbally, tend to understand and retain the video information better.

After showing the initial video to a patient, Dr. Volandes knew that the only way to roll out its use more widely was to develop a randomized trial of the video, and a study involving 50 cancer patients. A later study by the research team involved 150 patients with different types of advanced cancer. Other studies were done with patients with different illnesses, including dementia, and in different settings, such as nursing homes.

"The research suggests that patients make better-informed decisions using a video because they see possible procedures and interventions with their own eyes," he wrote. Moreover, the videos inspire patients to have what Dr. Volandes calls The Conversation with their doctors. [10]

Currently, the videos are only available for health care systems to use for patient education—physicians toting laptops or tablets can access the videos wherever their patients are—although the acpdecisions.org website does offer resources and checklists for patients and their families.

How Doctors Choose

Education is a continuing process. There may be no better way to learn than to spend decades treating patients. Observing how oftentimes aggressive and ultimately futile treatment can make patients' final days go terribly awry can affect how physicians feel about how they envision their own ends. It is instructive to know what their own treatment preferences are.

Between 1948 and 1964, the Johns Hopkins University School of Medicine signed up 1,337 physicians in graduating classes as volunteers to regularly fill out detailed questionnaires about their health, their lives, and their habits over the decades that followed. The Precursors Study, as the research

Last Comforts

is called, was originally envisioned as a way of determining risk factors for a variety of diseases, particularly heart disease. However, it has morphed into a study of aging itself.

Dr. Joe Gallo of Johns Hopkins spoke to reporter Sean Cole in a Radiolab podcast on "The Bitter End" in January 2013, Hopkins researchers, beginning in 1998, started asking the physicians who were then in their sixties, seventies, and eighties, how they wanted to die. More specifically, they were asked which kinds of treatments they would want, assuming they had limited brain function, didn't recognize those close to them, and couldn't speak. Symptoms, in other words, like severe dementia. They were given a list of 10 possible treatments, which reminded me of the 10 plagues in Egypt that we recite every Passover: CPR, ventilation, dialysis, chemotherapy, surgery, invasive testing, feeding tube, blood transfusions, antibiotics, IV hydration, and pain medication.

With the exception of pain medication, [11] the physicians said they would choose none of the above. Ninety percent said no to CPR. Almost as many said no to ventilation and dialysis. Eighty percent said no surgery and no invasive tests, while nearly 80 percent said no feeding tube or blood products. Sixty percent said no to IV hydration.

A more recent study from the Stanford University School of Medicine echoed the results of the Precursors Study: in 2013, it found that 88.3 percent of nearly 2,000 physicians surveyed said they would choose "no-code" or do-not-resuscitate orders for themselves. [12]

Educating Physicians to Talk the Talk

People outside of the medical profession might not have become aware of the Precursors Study, had it not been for an essay called "How Doctors Die" that Ken Murray, MD (then Clinical Assistant Professor of Family Medicine at University of Southern California) published in 2011 at Zócalo Public Square, a non-profit ideas exchange. Doctors tend to seek less aggressive end-of-life care than ordinary patients do, he wrote, because they know when further treatment is likely to be futile and when they would consider life to no longer be worth living. [13]

A "tsunami broke out after it was published," Dr. Murray declared during the Radiolab podcast, where he participated with Dr. Gallo. The essay garnered thousands of comments—many of them from anguished family members still angry and aggrieved over their loved ones' difficult deaths. It also generated much news coverage and was translated into several languages. When Ezra Klein of the *Washington Post* challenged Dr. Murray over whether there was real proof behind his assertions, Dr. Murray wrote a follow-up, which he described as a kind of "endnotes" to his essay, in the *Wall Street Journal*.

"A lot of times we do things to people that we wouldn't do to a terrorist," he said, citing the need to sedate patients to the point of paralysis in order to connect them to a ventilator. The patients are not asleep, but they are completely helpless, he added.

Last Comforts

When Dr. Murray was in practice as a family physician, he routinely asked any patient of his over 50, "How do you want to die?" Not surprisingly, his patients may have been surprised by the question, particularly if they were in good health, but it gave them food for thought. Their answers gave Dr. Murray a better sense of how best to care for them.

"Patients were universally grateful that I asked the question," he said during the podcast.

I would be too, if my doctor ever asks me.

Chapter 9 Endnotes

1. Angelo Volandes, MD. *The Conversation: A Revolutionary Plan for End-of-Life Care*. New York: Bloomsbury USA, 2015.

2. Committee on Approaching Death, Institute of Medicine. *Dying in America: Improving Quality and Honoring Individual Preferences Near the End of Life*. Washington, DC: The National Academies Press, 2015.

3. This is what the LCME calls for: (www.LCME.org): 7.2 Organ Systems/Life Cycle/Primary Care/Prevention/ Wellness/Symptoms/ Signs/ Differential Diagnosis, Treatment Planning, Impact of Behavioral/Social Factors

The faculty of a medical school ensure that the medical curriculum includes content and clinical experiences related to each organ system; each phase of the human life cycle; continuity of care; and preventive, acute, chronic, rehabilitative, end-of-life, and primary care in order to prepare students to:

—Recognize wellness, determinants of health, and opportunities for health promotion and disease prevention.

—Recognize and interpret symptoms and signs of disease.

—Develop differential diagnoses and treatment plans.

—Recognize the potential health-related impact on patients of behavioral and socioeconomic factors.

—Assist patients in addressing health-related issues involving all organ systems.

Chapter 9 Endnotes

4. Mary Ann Liebert, Inc. "Palliative Care in Medical School Curricula: A Survey of United States Medical Schools" *Journal of Palliative Medicine*, 11:9, 2008.

5. Mary Ann Liebert, Inc. "The Impact of a Clinical Rotation in Hospice: Medical Students' Perspectives." *Journal of Palliative Medicine*. 14:1, 2011.

6. National Palliative Care Registry. Comparative Performance Reports https://registry.capc.org/cms/Reports.aspx

7. D. Lupu. "Estimate of current hospice and palliative medicine workforce shortage." *Journal of Pain and Symptom Management* 2010 Dec. 40(6): 899–911.

8. W.F. Baile, R. Buckman, R. Lenzi, G. Glober, E.A. Beale, A.P. Kudelka. "SPIKES-A six-step protocol for delivering bad news: application to the patient with cancer." *Oncologist*. 2000. 5(4):302–1.
theoncologist.alphamedpress.org/content/5/4/302.full

9. The VitalTalk "talking maps" are at www.vitaltalk.org. The VitalTalk app is available at iTunes.

10. Patients learn and retain information better from watching instructive videos than from getting information verbally. Randomized, controlled trial of a video decision-support tool for cardiopulmonary resuscitation decision making in advanced cancer. *Journal of Clinical Oncology*. Jan. 31, 2013. jco.ascopubs.org/content/31/3/380.full.pdf+html

Chapter 9 Endnotes

11. Gallo, J.J., JB Straton, M. J. Klag, L.A. Meoni, D.P. Sulmasy, N-Y Wang, and D.E. Ford, "Life-sustaining treatments: What do physicians want and do they express their wishes to others?" *Journal of the American Geriatrics Society* 51(7), 961–9. 2003.
https://www.youtube.com/watch?v=m6e4_Guqsew

12. med.stanford.edu/news/all-news/2014/05/most-physicians-would-forgo-aggressive-treatment-for-themselves-.html

13. Dr. Kenneth Murray's original article about how doctors die: www.zocalopublicsquare.org/2011/11/30/how-doctors-die/ideas/nexus/
http://thehealthcareblog.com/blog/2012/08/29/doctors-really-do-die-differently/

10

The Nursing Perspective: The Heart of Care

 It is through the hands, the voice, the work of nursing that we can transform the end of life into a profound, sacred, healing experience."—Betty Ferrell, professor and research scientist, City of Hope National Medical Center, Los Angeles. [1]

For a brief time one winter, and to provide a respite for his live-in aide, I visited Frank, who was in his 80s and living in his monastic apartment in a public housing building in a riverfront town. The living room was bare except for Frank in his hospital bed and the TV on a stand near the door of the apartment's balcony. The floor was bare, too, so the sound of his oxygen machine echoed throughout the room. Pictures of children at various ages decorated one wall; I never learned if they were his children, his grandchildren, nieces, or nephews. "Debility and decline" was his diagnosis. Mostly, he slept, though once he awoke as I sat by his bedside to let him know I was there, opened his eyes briefly, looked as if he was alarmed, then fell back to sleep.

He mostly slept when his hospice nurse visited him, too, which didn't stop her from greeting him as warmly as an old friend. She talked gently to him, but loudly enough for him to hear. Her affection for this man seemed to flow from her as she checked his vitals. Her focus was intense but calm, almost meditative. It was a moment of great intimacy. And it was not the only time that the practice of nursing struck me as the being the heart and soul of palliative and hospice care. Or seeing that healing can go far beyond the conventional notion of "cure."

"I love him," she whispered to me, squeezing his hand before she left. "He's my favorite."

❧❧

No other health professionals spend as much time providing hands-on care for the sick than nurses. And perhaps because of a deep connection to patients' bodies and spirits woven into this care, it often falls to nurses to engage in difficult and ongoing conversations with patients and their families about the realities of their illness, when physicians have not done so, or when the families have been too overwhelmed

The Nursing Perspective

to hear what physicians have said.

The origins of hospice care, in fact, lie in nursing. Dame Cicely Saunders, who founded hospice as we know it now, had been a nurse before she became a physician. And she became a physician because it meant that she would be taken more seriously as she pursued her goal of opening a hospital outside of London to relieve the physical, emotional, psychological and spiritual suffering of those with terminal illnesses.

And it was a nurse who was instrumental in bringing hospice to the U.S. In 1965, two years after Saunders had given a lecture at Yale University about specialized care for the dying, Florence Wald, who was Dean of the Yale School of Nursing at the time, invited Saunders to become a visiting faculty member of the school for the spring term. In 1968, Wald took a sabbatical from Yale to work at St. Christopher's, the hospice Saunders had opened the year before. In 1974, Wald along with two pediatricians and a chaplain founded the first hospice in the U.S., now known as Connecticut Hospice in Branford, Connecticut.

It has been nurses, too, who have led the way in filling the gaps in educating the profession's current and future generations about end-of-life care.

Why has that been necessary? How are nurses educated to care for our most vulnerable populations? Nursing curricula, like medical school curricula, still leave something to be desired in terms of education in end-of-life care. Since 2008, according to the Institute of Medicine, baccalaureate nursing programs are required to include end-of-life care, but the average time devoted to the subject was under 15 hours.

In a study of nursing education called "ACE.S: Advancing Care Excellence for Seniors," the John A. Hartford Foundation noted:

"Unfortunately, most nurses, like most other health professionals, have traditionally received little education in the care of older adults," It cited a 2008 survey showing that geriatric content amounted to 10 to 25 percent of the content across all courses in most associate degree nursing programs—and that this content was rarely presented by faculty members who specialized in geriatrics. [2]

According to the National League for Nursing, more than half of all Registered Nurses receive their initial education in associate degree programs, including half of all nurses working in nursing homes or extended-care facilities. Nursing is becoming increasingly important in primary care and chronic care, particularly as care shifts away from hospitals and toward the home, community, or long-term care setting. Because this directly affects so many of us, it matters quite a lot that there is little formal education in the care of older adults, or in end-of life care. [3]

Actually, using the term "nurse" is somewhat incomplete because there is a huge range of educational paths, degrees, and certifications in the nursing profession. To become a registered nurse, a student can pursue a two-year program leading to an Associate Degree in Nursing (ADN). The student can then become a licensed practical nurse or a licensed vocational nurse. Or, there are hospital diploma programs and four-year, baccalaureate-level Bachelor of Science in Nursing

The Nursing Perspective

(BSN) programs. These programs are classified as pre-licensure nursing education. [4]

At the more advanced end of the education spectrum, the National Board for Certification of Hospice and Palliative Nurses offers seven different specialty certifications in palliative care. Advanced certified hospice and palliative nurses, those with the most training in this field, are nurse practitioners or clinical nurse specialists who deliver care similar to that delivered by physician specializing in hospice and palliative medicine.

More than 300 institutions offer doctoral nursing programs in the U.S. The PhD programs prepare nurses to become investigative researchers and to disseminate their findings, aimed at advancing the practice of nursing; the Doctor of Nursing Practice programs prepare nurses to become leaders in interdisciplinary health care teams and to translate evidence gained through nursing research into practice.

One of the most ambitious and effective programs to improve nursing education in palliative care is the End-of-Life Nursing Education Consortium (ELNEC) project.

Launched nationally to improve end-of-life care by nurses, it was founded on the premise that nurses cannot practice what they do not know. It was designed to train undergraduate and graduate nursing educators as well as those who teach in the profession's continuing education and staff development programs. Nursing leaders in palliative care serve as faculty for these train-the-trainer courses. Administered by the American Association of Colleges of Nursing (AACN) in Washington DC and the City of Hope National Medical Center in Los Angeles, it began in February 2000 with a grant from the Robert Wood Johnson Foundation.

Each ELNEC core curriculum consists of eight modules: an overview; pain management; symptom management; ethical/legal issues; cultural considerations in end-of-life care; communication; loss, grief, and bereavement; and preparation for, and care at the time of death and the final hour. ELNEC Core was the first curriculum developed. It was followed by specialized curricula for critical care, geriatric, pediatric, advanced-practice registered nurse, and for veterans. ELNEC has also developed a special curriculum for public hospitals in California.

Since ELNEC's original five-year funding from the Robert Wood Johnson Foundation, the project gained additional funding support from the National Cancer Institute, Open Society, Aetna, Archstone, Oncology Nursing Society, Bristol-Myers Squibb, Milbank, Cambia Health, California Healthcare Foundation, and the U.S. Department of Veterans Affairs.

More than 19,500 nurses and other health-care providers have attended ELNEC train-the-trainer courses. ELNEC trainers have returned to their institutions and communities and trained about 550,000 nurses and other health-care providers. ELNEC courses are also available online through Relias Learning. Originally envisioned as a United States project, ELNEC has gone international and its curriculum presented in 85 countries on six continents in eight languages.

For anyone who wants to learn about palliative nurs-

The Nursing Perspective

ing care or ELNEC, all roads lead to Betty Ferrell. A professor and research scientist at City of Hope in Los Angeles, Dr. Ferrell began her oncology nursing career in 1977 when most people were unfamiliar with the words "hospice" and "palliative care." In the interim decades, she has become the authority and guiding light for those practicing and aspiring to practice in the field. She's written eight books, including co-editing the first and subsequent editions of the Oxford Textbook of Palliative Nursing with her friend Nessa Coyle, a pioneer in palliative care at Memorial Sloan Kettering. She has written for more than 300 peer-reviewed publications, and she has been honored for her work numerous times.

Dr. Ferrell's steady, methodical approach, coupled with compassion and droll humor, make her a notable advocate. She is a member of the board of scientific advisors of the National Cancer Institute and she chairs the National Consensus Project for Quality Palliative Care. With a profound conviction about the importance of understanding spirituality at the end of life, Dr. Ferrell earned a master's degree in theology, ethics, and culture from Claremont Graduate University in 2007.

ELNEC had its origins in the 1990s with Dr. Ferrell's research on how nurses were trained in pain management and the broader issues of life-limiting illnesses. It became apparent that better nursing education was needed. When she sought funding to pursue that in 1997, she and her colleagues at first faced "nothing but closed doors."

Then, the Robert Wood Johnson Foundation stepped in with a grant to study nursing textbooks, licensing exams, and the attitudes and knowledge base of students and nurses.

"The results were overwhelming," Ferrell said.

The study showed that less than two percent of content in nursing textbooks was related to end-of-life care, and nursing faculty had very limited knowledge in teaching such care.

After the study results were published, the Robert Wood Johnson Foundation provided the initial grant to develop the End-of-Life Nursing Education Consortium, which has come to be known by its acronym, ELNEC. With new funding, Dr. Ferrell recalled, "Five of us sat down at a table with blank paper and we said, now what do we do? What do we teach? It was a bit scary. There's so much to teach."

The original ELNEC course (ELNEC-Core) was a train-the-trainer program that lasted three days. It featured lectures, role playing, small group, and case-study discussions, and networking opportunities.

Dr. Ferrell and her staff and faculty continuously evaluate the course work. They update the curriculum annually. ELNEC participants are asked to rate the courses based on 20 criteria. They also document support for disseminating the curriculum from their nursing school dean and they report back to the ELNEC project on the ways the curriculum is subsequently implemented. That's a way to maintain program integrity and to learn what impact it is having.

In 2014, the trainers who took ELNEC courses in turn conducted about 250 courses in their own institutions.

"It's like the greatest pyramid scheme," Dr. Ferrell joked. More seriously, she added, "Great things are happening. We have many messengers, which is good because the needs are enormous.

"We get a 4.9 mean rating [out of a possible 5] and we say, OK now we need to change everything," Dr. Ferrell said. "Our overworked staff asks, 'are you kidding? When are you going to stop?'

And the answer seems to be, not any time soon.

"We're always fine-tuning."

What guides them, besides the body of evidence amassing in the field of palliative care and the desire to keep their curriculum connected to the real world in which nurses practice daily? It is that Dr. Ferrell, and her team, define palliative care as the kind of care they want for themselves and for the people they love.

Dr. Ferrell is encouraged that palliative care is increasingly integrated into routine care, in fields such as cardiology, pulmonology, dementia, and long-term care. She is a self-described optimist.

"When we used to read stories about difficult deaths, or witness them, we used to think, that's how it is. Now we know it doesn't have to be that way. We know what superb care looks like."

The bad news, though, is that with palliative care moving into the mainstream of health care, she believes it has morphed from a passionate, spiritual movement into one focused on immediate medical issues.

"Pain and symptom management isn't palliative care."

It is time, she said, to advocate for real palliative care, which is interdisciplinary and includes a strong spiritual component. Spiritual distress needs to be treated the same as any other medical problem.

"If you're not providing good spiritual care, you're not providing good palliative care."

Dr. Ferrell is not necessarily referring to religion. In 2009, a Consensus Conference sponsored by the Archstone Foundation gathered 40 leaders from the realms of palliative care and spiritual care to address the issue of improving the quality of spiritual care as a dimension of palliative care. Ferrell shared leadership of the conference. The subsequent report was published in the *Journal of Palliative Medicine,* with Christina Puchalski, MD, of the George Washington Institute for Spirituality and Health. [5] One of the remarkable things that emerged from the conference was that 40 strong-minded individuals could actually agree on a definition of spirituality. Here it is:

"Spirituality is the aspect of humanity that refers to the way individuals seek and express meaning and purpose and the way they experience their connectedness to the moment, to self, to others, to nature and to the significant or sacred."

Dr. Ferrell believes that spiritual distress must be treated the same as any other medical problem and that spiritual care must be incorporated into the goals of care that are developed for patients.

Are nurses who care for the elderly, the frail, the chronically ill, and the dying a self-selecting group whose in-

The Nursing Perspective

ner compasses point them in a particular direction? Can kindness and compassion be taught? I was fortunate to have an opportunity to pose those questions and more to six ELNEC leaders, doctorates all, and each coming from wildly different backgrounds.

Pam Malloy is director of the ELNEC project. She had been an oncology nurse for 25 years. When ELNEC had one year left on its initial grant, a representative of the American Association of Colleges of Nursing called to find out whether she would consider directing ELNEC. At the time, Dr. Malloy was head of education at George Washington Hospital. She supervised 2,500 people.

One year? "I thought I could do that," she told me. More than a dozen years later, she continues in the role, for which she said she is both passionate and grateful.

When ELNEC received its original funding, Dr. Malloy said, "We were naïve. We thought we'd be done [in the five years of the RWJF grant] and have everyone trained by then." It did not work out that way. One unexpected but beneficial development is that physicians, social workers, pharmacists, financial officers, and chaplains have attended the courses, enriching the curriculum.

Are nurses who practice end-of-life care a self-selecting group?

While many describe it as a calling, Dr. Malloy says it is more germane that these nurses are "astute and attuned to the people they're caring for."

Dr. Patricia Berry started her career after graduating from the College of St. Teresa in Winona, Minnesota with a

181

Last Comforts

Bachelor of Science in 1973. She was interested in oncology at a time when, as she put it, "nothing was curable." She worked with a nurse manager, who had cancer and taught Dr. Berry and her nursing colleagues how to care for her as she was dying.

Now a tenured associate professor at the University of Utah Hartford Center of Geriatric Nursing Excellence, Dr. Berry is certified as an advanced practice palliative care nurse.

Before joining the faculty at the University of Utah, she oversaw the collaboration between the University of Wisconsin and the Joint Commission on the Accreditation of Healthcare Organizations, which produced pain assessment and management standards. Dr. Berry keeps framed pictures of memorable former patients above her desk.

"They showed me what it was like to live, as they died."

Dr. Berry has seen a change in nursing students over the years and sees a more balanced approach to matters of life and death in successive generations of nurses.

"You can talk about death in polite company. I used to lie about what I did. I didn't want to make people uncomfortable."

Dr. Carol Long, who appeared in Chapter 4 discussing care for dementia patients, believes insufficient attention is paid to palliative care in nursing homes.

Of nursing education, she said, "We need to do a better job at the undergraduate level."

The ELNEC-Geriatric curriculum was designed to provide advanced training for geriatric nurses who work in

The Nursing Perspective

long-term care and skilled nursing facilities, and in the hospices that service these facilities. The curriculum includes strategies for training unlicensed personnel, such as certified nursing assistants (CNAs) who work with geriatric patients and their families. The challenge with this curriculum, Betty Ferrell said, is the difficulty in getting trainers from nursing facilities to travel to where ELNEC training occurs.

Dr. Barbara Head, assistant professor of medicine and director of the Interdisciplinary Program for Palliative Care and Chronic Illness at the University of Louisville, has taught the ELNEC geriatric curriculum nationally. With a masters in social work, she began her career working with adolescents and elders in nursing homes. After her mother's experience as a hospice patient, Dr. Head became a hospice social worker and later went to nursing school.

She worked at the Hospice of Louisville for 11 years as a home hospice nurse, director of quality improvement, and director of education. She was awarded her doctoral degree at 53, and became research director at the university, administering grants in palliative care.

"Most palliative care nurses, physicians, and social workers are passionate about what they do because it is holistic and meaningful," she said. As for nursing and medical school students, she said, they often do not understand exactly what palliative care and hospice care are and how they work together. They are surprised that symptom management can be addressed long before the end of life. Some go into a clinical rotation "thinking it will be the most depressing week of their lives, and they're surprised by how upbeat and caring

183

the practitioners are. They get attached to the patients and families they see."

Students may also believe that it is unprofessional to show emotion in caring for the very ill, but Dr. Head reassures them that "It's okay to feel and to cry, as long as it's not about you. Otherwise, we're setting [the students] up to be robots."

Some students say, "I could never do this" as a career, but others tell her "This is how I envisioned medicine when I went to school." One advantage that today's students have is that "The science of palliative care has really advanced. We know so much more about symptom management."

Dr. Head teaches an online course in death and grief, enabling her to reach more students at the School of Social Work. Her students—the digital generation—love using an online textbook and seeing contemporary films. She said they can learn good communication and listening skills in these ways.

Dr. Marian Grant, assistant professor at the University of Maryland School of Nursing, is a nurse practitioner certified in palliative and acute care. In Baltimore, she volunteered with an AIDS hospice in the early 1990s, and found the experience profound. A marketing and advertising professional at Procter and Gamble for 20 years, she pursued her second career as a nurse.

"One hundred years ago, people died at home. You couldn't get out of childhood without being exposed to it," she said. "Now people die in institutions and it's unusual for more than the immediate family to be present. So students don't know what this process looks like."

Dr. Grant has been teaching nursing students since 2005. After a lecture, she often hears student comments like "This is what I went to nursing school for."

Students recognize that they don't get enough training, she said.

"People have an abiding wish not to be dead; that's insurmountable."

Dr. Grant is hopeful that palliative care will become more widely acceptable to the public "before we get to the death part."

Dr. Kathi Lindstrom, assistant professor at the Vanderbilt University School of Nursing, teaches palliative care courses for Doctor of Nursing Practice and Master of Science in Nursing programs. She said she's "on a mission to have a good death for everyone."

With three careers behind her, Dr. Lindstrom went to nursing school at 40. In addition to teaching, she sees homebound patients as part of the House Calls program, connected with the Clinic at Mercury Court in the Vanderbilt School of Nursing. Like Marian Grant, Dr. Lindstrom has spent considerable time with geriatric and AIDS patients. Her practice is informed by personal experience. Her father has suffered from dementia for 10 years.

Are her students a self-selecting group?

"Absolutely," she replied while emphasizing that compassion and a sense of calling are not enough. Skill building and practice are critical. The average age of her students is 22.

One student, not atypically, told her, "My grandma died an awful death and I went into [palliative care] to change this."

Training Advanced Care Workers

By 2050, 27 million of us will need some form of long-term care. That's more than double the number in 2010, according to the Milken Institute School of Public Health at George Washington University. The need will require an army of direct care workers—including certified nursing assistants, home health aides, and personal care aides. That army will help us bathe, get dressed, eat, go to the bathroom, move safely from one place to another (whether that is from wheelchair to bed, room to room, or out for a walk) and get tucked comfortably back in bed at night. The aides will keep a watchful eye on us to note possibly troubling changes in mood, physical well-being, or mental functioning. It can be difficult, physically taxing work requiring strength, patience, and presence of mind in the face of unexpected events or crises.

And yet, ironically, providing direct care to our population's most vulnerable people requires the least amount of training. The work experiences the highest turnover rate—and pays the least—of the caring professions. Requirements vary from state to state, but certified nursing assistants must typically attend 40 hours of training, serve a supervised 'externship,' and pass an exam to be certified. No formal education is required for home health and personal care aides,

186

The Nursing Perspective

but those working in certified home-health or hospice agencies must get formal training, typically 75 hours, and pass a standard test. As the Institute of Medicine noted in its 2008 report Retooling for an Aging America: Building the Health-care Workforce, your dog groomer requires more training than that. Clearly, there is a disconnect here.

There is also a disconnect between the current size of the direct-care workforce and the numbers needed as the aging population grows. The U.S. Bureau of Labor Statistics estimated there were more than 3.5 million direct care workers in 2012. Projected demand calls for an additional 1.3 million new positions by 2022. Most aides will be needed in home or community-based settings, not in long-term care facilities. PHI, the Paraprofessional Healthcare Institute, projects that by 2022 home and community workers will outnumber those in facilities by a ratio of two to one. [6]

Inadequate training and lack of supervision—at all levels of government, not to mention within the home health care industry itself—has certainly opened the door to egregious cases of elder abuse, neglect, and fraud by aides. However, my intent here is not to focus on the many considerable red flags that bear watching in hiring or in managing direct care workers for ourselves or for our loved ones, but to point to a few ways that certain organizations are working to improve the quality of such care.

Following the IOM's report on the health care workforce, the Eldercare Workforce Alliance (EWA), a group of 30 national organizations, representing all aspects of inter-disciplinary care, family caregivers, and consumers, joined together to address the immediate and future workforce crisis in caring for an aging America and to recommend practical solutions.

"By 2020, you won't be able to be a health care provider and not deal with older adults," Caitlin Connolly said. When we spoke, she was the EWA project director. "We need to attract more people in the pipeline, so we have the faculty and trainers to train the workforce."

What will it take to enable every worker to operate at his or her highest level of skills? What should be the scope of practice? Focusing on the issue of care in the home setting, EWA convened several roundtable discussions between November 2010 and June 2013. One included asking ten direct-care workers for their views on such questions as what they feel comfortable doing; what kind of training and supervision is appropriate; how they wanted to participate with an interdisciplinary team; and how communication with families and health care providers could be encouraged.

Connolly said that the participants identified a number of skills they wanted to work on, including palliative and end-of-life care. They wanted to be better trained in preventive measures, as well as in dealing with dementia. EWA also held roundtable discussions with nurses, physicians, and social workers and conducted a survey of family caregivers.

Because of these discussions and surveys, EWA concluded that there should be a new, higher designation in direct care, that of the Advanced Direct Care Worker (ADCW) position. As a respected member of a comprehensive team, the ADCW would support a care plan set by a nurse, physician, and social worker. With the right training, supervision, and model of care, EWA believes that advanced direct care workers could provide better quality care and communication with patient families and they could support pain management. Depending on state regulations, and with proper training, they could also administer medications.

Eldercare Workforce Alliance co-convenor Nancy Lundebjerg said, "We were very clear about the guidelines that needed to be there." That would include the extra level of training to develop more sophisticated skills, the necessity of observing, recording, and reporting any changes in a patient's status, such as cognitive changes, or changes in appetite or weight.

"We want to make sure that advanced skills and responsibilities translate into increased wages," Lundebjerg said.

EWA developed the concept of advanced direct care workers because "We wanted to do something at the national level," Lundebjerg said. From a practical perspective and for the idea to become reality, it would have to be rolled out state by state.

The Eldercare Workforce Alliance is hoping that, in the next decade, a career ladder will be developed that sets a standard for wages and benefits, and provides an opportunity for advancement. A career path, along with improved wages and benefits, are needed to keep workers in the field. In the meantime, EWA encourages state certification agencies to increase competency-training standards for direct-care workers, with a minimum requirement of 120 hours of training that includes geriatric-care content. Along with training for certified nursing assistants and home health aides, EWA advocates creating minimum training standards for non-clinical, direct-care workers, such as personal care attendants. [7]

❧❧

In Springdale, Arkansas, the Schmieding Center for Senior Health and Education had long been involved in training family caregivers and direct care workers to better care for the frail and the ill. In 2012, the Centers for Medicare & Medicaid Innovation Center awarded the center a $3.6 million grant for cost-effective delivery of enhanced home caregiver training.

The Schmieding Center was established in January 1999 as the first satellite center on aging affiliated with the Donald W. Reynolds Institute on Aging at the University of Arkansas for Medical Sciences. A primary reason behind benefactor Lawrence Schmieding's gift was to develop a home-caregiver training program because, as he put it, "where there's home there's hope."

The center has been offering caregiving workshops since 2001. Its certified caregiver program has trained thousands of direct care workers and family caregivers. Dr. Larry Wright, geriatrician and the center director, told me that when they set out to create the curriculum, they sought role models.

"We searched for six months, and there were no good examples so we put together our own curriculum," he said.

Contrary to the view that direct care workers in a home setting do not require the same training as those who

The Nursing Perspective

work in an institution, Dr. Wright believes they need more. One disadvantage for workers in the home setting is that there are no policies and procedures in place. Aides are sometimes called upon to make decisions for which they might not be prepared. That is addressed in 116 hours of training for physical and cognitive skills and health literacy.

In making this grant, the Centers for Medicare and Medicaid Services (CMS) noted that better quality care in the home leads to "fewer avoidable hospital admissions and readmissions, better preventive care, better compliance with care and avoidance of unnecessary institutional care." Over a three-year period, the grant was to support training of an estimated 2,100 workers in Arkansas, California, Hawaii, and Texas, through online, distance learning.

When applying for the CMS grant, agency leaders considered what would be innovative and make a difference. Dr. Wright said the answer was to provide advanced training for aides so they could become family-care advocates. That meant adding a 40-hour module to its basic home caregiver training.

The grant gave the center the ability to convert its curriculum for online access. The key to getting the grant, in Dr. Wright's view, was building in a program for micro-credit loans in each state to cover tuition costs and recruitment efforts. It was a way to attract people to this workforce.

"We think these [home health] aides are underused and under-appreciated by the health care system," he said. "We wanted them to have adequate communication skills and knowledge about chronic illnesses, the disease trajectory, and what their role can be." In short, the goal is to create person-centered care in which aides can better understand the elders in their care, including what quality of life means to them.

For family caregivers, Dr. Wright said, the classes emphasize the importance of recognizing how stressful and energy-depleting these responsibilities can be.

"People tend to underestimate the toll caregiving takes," he said. Most helpful for caregivers is to learn the course of an illness—a road map—and to have the resources to stay on path and not feel isolated.

For caregivers who cannot attend classes, the center developed a DVD set called ElderStay@home Home Caregiving Skills for Families. It comes with a companion booklet based on its unique curriculum. The set covers 57 "Watch & Do" basic, intermediate, and advanced home-caregiving skills. (A link to the set is on the Center's web site.) [8]

Dr. Wright freely admits that since 1999, nearly everything he's learned about caregiving has come from working at the center, and from working with nurses. He recognizes "This is one piece of a very complex puzzle. I continue to be increasingly aware that when you swim in a system that's all about acute care, it's hard to focus on other issues that are just as important."

Are there any settings in which certified nursing assistants are learning and practicing the kinds of advanced skills advocated by EWA and taught by the Schmieding Center? Are there settings where CNAs are working as respected and important members of teams of health care practitioners? The answer is yes, and the following chapter on nursing home transformation shows how it is done.

Chapter 10 Endnotes

1. Betty Ferrell, in a keynote speech accepting the Episteme Award by the nursing honor society, Sigma Theta Tau, at its Biennial Convention, Nov. 18, 2013. The Episteme Award, supported by the Baxter International Foundation, is given to a nurse who has contributed significantly to nursing knowledge development, application, or discovery that results in a recognizable and sizable benefit to the public.

2. www.jhartfound.org/images/uploads/reports/150212b_NLN_ACES_Report.pdf

3. Report on ACE.S: Advancing Care Excellence for Seniors: Reflections on a Nursing Education Program funded by the John A. Hartford Foundation.

4. www.jhartfound.org/images/uploads/reports/150212b_NLN_ACES_Report.pdf

5. P. Ironside, E. Tagliareni, B. McLaughlin, E. King, A. Mengel (2010). "Fostering Geriatrics in Associate Degree Nursing Education: An Assessment of Current Curricula and Clinical Experiences." Journal of Nursing Education, 49, 246–52

6. Report on nursing curricula, referenced in J. Hartford Foundation report on ACE.S www.nln.org/aboutnln/livingdocuments/pdf/nlnvision_7.pdf

7. "A Vision for Recognition of the Role of Licensed Practical/Vocational Nurses in Advancing the Nation's Health: A Living Document from the National League for Nursing (NLN) Board of Governors," September 2014. ACE.S was

the first national effort to prepare students in all pre-licensure nursing programs, including associate degree, to deliver high-quality care to older adults. The original Hartford grant, Fostering Geriatrics in Associate Degree Nursing Education (2007–09), led to a second grant, known as ACE.S (2007–12). The National League for Nursing (NLN) and Community College of Philadelphia (CCP) led ACE.S, under the direction of Elaine Tagliareni, EdD, RN, CNE, FAAN. She was then both president of the NLN and a professor of nursing at CCP. She was next appointed NLN's chief program officer. See more at: www.jhartfound.org/blog/for-improving-the-nursing-care-of-older-adults-its-ace-s-in-my-book/

8. https://smhs.gwu.edu/gwish/about

9. http://phinational.org/files/phi-factsheet14update-12052014.pdf

10. http://www.eldercareworkforce.org/issues-and-solutions/workforce-shortage/issue:workforce-shortage/

11. www.schiedingcenter.org/caregiverproducts.html

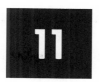

Nursing Home Transformation

"Nursing homes based on the medical model are not the best environment for long-term care."—Ray Rusin, retired as chief of the office of health facility regulation for the Rhode Island Department of Health. [1]

What is it about the idea of nursing homes that makes people cringe? Is it the affront of bad smells in rooms and hallways? Images of neglect or mistreatment at the hands of indifferent staff? Or the unsettling image of frail, demented and disconsolate elders lined up in the halls in their wheelchairs, with those thousand-yard stares, like something out of a bad zombie movie?

I've visited people in five of the nursing homes that Holy

Last Comforts

Name Medical Center contracts with in Bergen County, New Jersey. They run the gamut from small and frayed around the edges to large, sunny, and gleaming. (Appearance does not necessarily indicate the quality of care inside.) I've never seen callousness, indifference, or cruelty from nurses and aides. Quite the contrary; I've seen much compassion, affection, and kindness, and this in spite of staffs being burdened with too much to handle in too little time and for what is likely too little compensation.

So what has made me cringe?

First, the noise. TVs blaring from most rooms. Periodic and often unintelligible announcements over the PA system. The rumble of carts, bearing medication, rolling through hallways. Chair and bed alarms that squawk when someone, who cannot walk, tries to get out of a chair or bed. The chorus of residents screaming, pleading, imploring: Take me home! Get me out of here! I hate you! Nurse! The cacophony in a large, drab common room that, on first glance, resembles a junior high school cafeteria with wheelchairs.

And then there are the mattresses. For the bedridden considered to be at risk for falls, it is not uncommon to see portable mattresses placed on the floor next to their beds, which have been lowered to their lowest possible level, to cushion a possible fall.

There was this insight, shared by Eleanor, a happily chatty 94-year-old woman I visited weekly, who always held my hand and gave me the rundown on who was who and who did what in the common room where a few dozen residents spent many hours a day. She was often seated in her throne-like rolling chair next to an uncommunicative woman who would become agitated from time to time. Eleanor would reach over and pat the woman's shoulder or caress her arm, which seemed to comfort the woman.

"In this place, people don't touch each other," Eleanor told me, by way of criticism.

If current trends continue, it's entirely possible that one-quarter of us will die in nursing homes. In fact, the Patient-Centered Outcomes Research Institute (PCORI), a nonprofit non-governmental organization authorized by the Affordable Care Act in 2010, estimates that by 2020, as many as 40 percent of U.S. deaths will take place in skilled nursing facilities. [2]

Consequently, how nursing homes are designed and operated matters a great deal.

Can we improve the quality of life and care in skilled nursing facilities? My first inkling that we could came from spending times with the elder nuns at St. Michael Villa, described in Chapter 6. But I've since seen that a radical re-thinking of what it means to honor, respect, and nurture the frail elderly and the very ill has given rise to residences that offer the comfort of home without the sense of institutionalization.

Last Comforts

Patient-Centered Care and Culture Change

These two phrases – patient-centered care and culture change -- are critical in thinking about the future of caring for the frail elderly and for those with advanced illness. They are particularly critical in looking at long-term care settings.

Isn't "patient-centered" a superfluous phrase? After all, isn't medical and nursing care centered on you as a patient? Not necessarily. Institutional care centers operate on a medical model premised on the efficient running of the institution.

The Institute of Medicine (IOM)'s Integrative Medicine and Patient-Centered Care (2009) reported that the hallmark of patient-centered care is "to customize treatment recommendations and decision-making in response to patients' preferences and beliefs." It cites research showing that such care "leads to enhanced patient satisfaction, better outcomes, improved health status, and reduced utilization of care."

The Pioneer Network, a nonprofit organization created in 1997, describes itself as being dedicated to creating a culture of aging that is life-affirming, satisfying, humane and meaningful. It defines culture change as "the national movement for the transformation of older adult services, based on person-directed values and practices where the voices of elders and those working with them are considered and respected. Core, person-directed values are choice, dignity, respect, self-determination, and purposeful living."

Nursing Home Transformation

These are not new phenomena. Both have their origins in the Omnibus Reconciliation Act of 1987.

In 1986, a blue ribbon panel, selected by the Institute of Medicine, completed a report on "Improving the Quality of Care in Nursing Homes." This report made it clear, for the first time, that quality of life carries equal weight with quality of care. Congress used the findings to mandate enforceable, minimal quality of care standards for long-term care facilities.

At the heart of the legislation, called OBRA '87, is resident quality of life and quality of care, establishing uniform standards designed to promote resident rights and maximize resident quality of care and functioning. The law mandated that the Centers for Medicare & Medicaid Services (CMS) develop and issue regulations to implement the law, which it did in 1990. The regulations compelled nursing homes to focus on the inherent right of each resident to "attain and maintain his/her highest practicable physical, mental, and psychosocial well-being."

It was not long after OBRA '87 passed that Bill Thomas, MD, had his "Eureka" moment. Thomas—a high-energy, charismatic polymath, outstanding storyteller, author of five books and a tireless promoter of the importance of embracing elderhood—is one of the visionaries of the culture change movement.

"I'm a nursing home abolitionist," Dr. Thomas said when I interviewed him, as he's said to anyone who'd listen since 1989. He was 31 then, and fresh out of residency. He worked as the medical director of Chase Memorial, an 80-bed nursing home in New Berlin, New York. His encounter with a patient, who declared, "I'm so lonely!"while he treated her arm rash, was transformational. He realized that, for elders in a nursing home, the enemies are loneliness, isolation, and boredom. The way to combat that is to offer elders a rich life of engagement with nature, and of empowerment, by enabling them to make choices about the course of their days—including when they want to rise, to eat, and to conduct other daily activities.

Thus was the Eden Alternative born, which Thomas founded with his wife Jude.

At the time, Mary Jane Koren, MD, was the director of New York State's Bureau of Long Term Care, which oversees nursing home certification. She provided a small grant (despite her staff's serious doubts) to enable Chase Memorial to change the environment by bringing in parakeets for residents to care for, as well as assorted cats and dogs. They replaced the front lawn with an organic garden. Children from nearby schools visited.

At a gathering of the Long Term Care Community Coalition where she was honored in 2014, Dr. Koren recalled visiting the nursing home less than a year after those changes were implemented. She found the atmosphere had changed— the hum of conversation, no one slumped in wheelchairs by the nursing station, and a marked drop in the use of psychoactive medications, food waste, and the use of dietary supplements. [3]

"The place felt alive," she said.

Several years later, Thomas came to Dr. Koren with another idea: what if the management and operation of a

Nursing Home Transformation

long-term facility could be transformed, so that both residents and the nursing assistants who care for them could be empowered? He envisioned a facility with the management structure flattened, the environment focused more on "home" than on "nursing," and the medical and the clinical components transformed from master to servant.

Thomas thought a lot about what word to use to refer to the nursing assistants who provide most of the direct care to residents. There weren't any English words that did justice to what he had in mind, he told me. He discovered an ancient Persian word, "shahbaz," which means "royal falcon," and he created a parable about a compassionate bird who has the power of speech and who ultimately turns its relationship with a tyrannical king upside-down. (An excellent and entertaining fable, do find time to read it for yourself. [4])

Thomas loves the image of the falcon soaring overhead, "protecting you, sustaining you, and nurturing you."

The nursing assistants would become the "shahbazzim" who would be the midwives for elderhood, finding "the magic in [the] rhythm of daily life." They would be given the responsibility and authority (not to mention continuous education and training) to work in a self-directed way. Nursing assistants provide most of the direct care for elders in long-term care settings. Therefore, they are in the best position to establish trusting and compassionate relationships with their elders. Not coincidentally, they are also in the best position to observe any changes, for good or ill, in their elders' well-being.

Last Comforts

Building upon the principles of the Eden Alternative, Thomas developed the Green House® Project. A central nursing station? Gone. Long corridors with rooms on both sides? Gone. A strict hierarchy of leadership? Gone too. Green Houses offer a cluster of private rooms with private bathrooms around a large kitchen and communal dining and living area. There are no set times to rise, to dine, or to get ready for bed.

The first Green House Home was built in Tupelo, Mississippi in 2003. With substantial help from the Robert Wood Johnson Foundation, which provided a $10 million grant over a five-year period beginning in 2005, to launch these small nursing homes, the Green House Project has grown to include, at this writing, 160 homes in 27 states. Though most are located in suburban areas and resemble large, single-family homes, others are in multi-story buildings in cities.

The Green House is just one variant on the theme of alternative nursing facilities. Sometimes they're called "households" or "small houses." Their "neighborhoods" might include more than the 10 bedrooms usually found in the Green House developments, and the aides who assist residents may be referred to as "universal workers" rather than shahbazzim, but these developments are similarly distinguished for their person-centered care and culture change approach to operations and management.

The concept "creates some cognitive dissonance," Thomas said, because their space and the staff roles and relationships are so different from conventional nursing homes.

Nursing Home Transformation

Changing the culture and relationships is much harder than actually changing the physical space, he said, in an uncharacteristic understatement.

The wonderful aroma of eggs, bacon, and French toast fills the air at mid-morning when you enter one of two 17-person residential "neighborhoods" on the fourth floor of Tockwotton on the Waterfront, a five-story senior living residence overlooking the Seekonk River in East Providence, Rhode Island. The first thing you see in this "neighborhood" is not a nurses' station, but a modern, open kitchen with a snack bar and tables and chairs overlooking the river. It is light and clean and quiet. No one is shrieking. Carts aren't rumbling. A PA system isn't crackling with announcements.

Tockwotton on the Waterfront, which opened in January 2013, is a five-story, 156-unit nursing-and-assisted-living center that looks like a seaside resort. It is adjacent to Bold Point Park in the southern portion of the city's Waterfront District. The $52.2 million building replaced a 140-year-old building in Providence that initially served as the Home for Aged Women. Four women, determined to provide compassionate care for elderly, destitute women in the last chapters of their lives, opened it in 1856 in a single-family house.

Tockwotton has several components: assisted living apartments; "memory care" apartments; short-term rehabilitation rooms and 35 long-term care rooms in two "neighborhoods." The neighborhoods have been fully occupied since the building opened.

Last Comforts

While the building's exterior is handsome and modern, the interior is the revelation. Its design balances community and privacy for its residents. Natural light bathes public and private spaces throughout. Numerous gathering spaces, large and small, encourage all residents to socialize, participate in activities, exercise, use the beauty parlor or the library/computer room. Dining choices include small, casual cafes or a larger dining room.

The two "neighborhoods" for skilled nursing are a revelation, too. Residents have their own rooms, which they can decorate as they please, and private bathrooms. There is no central nurses' station. Medications are dispensed from small lockers in residents' rooms. Instead of institutional-looking rails along the halls, the rails look more like wainscoting that allow a person to lean on them for support, if needed. Each neighborhood has its own small laundry room where the nursing assistants do residents' laundry three times a week.

Technology is used unobtrusively here. The staff uses laptops or notebook computers, which they can work on in any of the airy and comfortable public spaces in the neighborhood. A computerized security system includes motion sensors in bathrooms and bedrooms that can detect a problem a resident might be having, such as incontinence or sleeplessness. When a problem is detected, the staff person's phone signals silently. If the staff person does not respond within a specific timeframe, the silent alarm rings a supervisor.

It took Tockwotton's founders just several days to open their home in 1856, but the gestation for Tockwotton

Nursing Home Transformation

on the Waterfront took more than a decade. Diane Dooley, who heads the senior living practice of the architecture firm DiMella Shaffer, said the firm had been working with Tockwotton for years, analyzing different sites, and when they wanted to relocate and expand. The waterfront site was a challenge, but its constraints proved also to be an advantage. It is linear but hilly, which enabled the architects to create access to the outdoors for residents from the building's first three levels. That access to garden and walkways—and having a hand in gardening—has been a boon for residents, particularly for elders in the memory-care section.

The architects' goal was to provide spaces that are livable, support independence, and offer a close connection to the outdoors, whether it is in a garden, a large porch, or by a view. It uses as much natural daylight as possible.

Tockwotton executive director Kevin McKay, who took me on a tour of the property, said, "We were doing culture change at the old Tockwotton," and they brought that culture change to the new facility.

McKay is a passionate advocate for consistent assignments—so nursing assistants and residents develop trusting relationships. He advocates self-organized work teams that meet regularly to review residents' status. He believes in the value of learning circles.

How do they work? He cited an example of a resident with some memory issues and occasional diarrhea. In a learning circle—in this case attended by a social worker, dietary staff member, nursing assistant and others—one person would present a problem and everyone would have a chance to speak uninterrupted, one at a time, in the circle. Solutions can arise from unexpected sources. Here, the dietary staff member made the simple but useful suggestion to cut back on the resident's prune juice, which he'd been drinking every day.

The struggle with this style of management, he admitted, is that it can take time for newly hired staff, more accustomed to the medical model of operations and management, to fully embrace culture change. It is also a challenge to find nursing assistants who can be equally skilled at housekeeping and cooking as they are at direct care. How would he advise others who might want to adopt the practices of culture change? Beyond the first major step, which would be for administration to buy into it, McKay said, "You can't do enough training."

Training is the hallmark for the shahbazzim at Green House Homes at Green Hill in West Orange, New Jersey.

Like Tockwotton, Green Hill's roots go back to the 19th century when the Society for the Relief of Respectable Aged Women opened a small residence for 13 women in Newark, New Jersey in 1866. It grew to house 60 elders, adding a nursing care unit in 1880. In 1958, the Society merged with the Newark YWCA, which had created a department for the incurable in its boarding house in 1881, added a second building a few years later, which they outgrew. They formed the Memorial Center for Women. In 1965, the board of directors purchased Green's Hotel, built in the 1920s in West Orange, New Jersey. (Fun fact: the building's grand exterior entry would be familiar to fans of "The Sopranos," as the nursing home to which Tony Soprano moved his mother.)

Nursing Home Transformation

In 1986, 33 new suites for assisted living were built on the site, and in 2011, two Green House Homes opened, the first Green House residences in New Jersey. The homes are stunning, single-level, arts-and-crafts style houses with welcoming porches and patios. Green Hill has approvals for two more homes on the site.

Toni Lynn Davis, president and CEO of Green Hill, is a third generation leader at this senior living community. Her mother had been president before her. Davis had worked here as a teen and took over the reins more than 10 years ago. She calls herself a "servant-leader."

As with Tockwotton in East Providence, Rhode Island, design of the Green House Homes is just the beginning of change. The certified nursing assistants are trained to be the shahbazzim. Ongoing training empowers them to make decisions about how the house runs. Two shahbazzim work during the day, two others work in the evening, and one is on duty overnight. There is a full array of group activities, including happy hour, and each house has its own rhythm, she said. These self-managed teams are accountable to each other. Nursing and specialty care, such as physical therapy, are available, but it's not a charge nurse at the head of a hierarchy of leadership here, she said. Perhaps not surprisingly, the Green House Homes have little staff turnover.

I asked a middle-aged man whose mother lives in one of the Green House Homes how his mother likes living there and what he thought of it. His mother is in her late '80s and has advanced dementia. She still knows her son, though not by name. He lives not far from Green Hill and sees her twice during the week plus visits on the weekend. He finds the home so welcoming that he has become friendly with the shahbazzim as well as families of other residents. He likes sitting by the fireplace when he visits. Sometimes he uses the kitchen too.

He likes that there are often activities such as games, arts and crafts, and pet therapy. He explained that his mother had been on antidepressants, but no longer takes them. Her blood pressure was elevated for a while but now is normal, without medication. She is always clean. He never feels anxious when he leaves.

"I feel privileged that she can live here," he said. "There's a lot of dignity for my Mom. To me she seems happy."

❧❧

I spoke with Adam Berman, president of the Chelsea Jewish Foundation, which provides all levels of senior living and services. In 2006, when the foundation wanted to build another nursing home on land it owned, Adam's father, CEO Barry Berman learned of and became captivated by the Green House concept. The nearly 95,000-square-foot Leonard Florence Center for Living in Chelsea, Massachusetts, which has been open since 2010, became the first urban, multi-story Green House development. Designed by DiMella Shaffer, the building houses 100 residents with 10 people living on each of 10 floors. Three "houses" serve people who need short-term rehabilitation. One "house" serves people living with ALS, a neurodegenerative disease. Another serves people with multiple sclerosis.

The building's first floor is its "Main Street," with a bakery, deli, spa, and chapel; each "house" also has its own communal area for games, social gatherings, and other events. Each "house" offers made-to-order Kosher meals. Residents and staff jointly design the menus.

During the planning process, as Adam Berman recalled, "We challenged ourselves to think of populations that are not served well by the traditional [long-term care] model," he said. "That included younger, disabled populations, such as those with ALS and MS." The foundation began reaching out to local organizations to learn what those populations needed and they confirmed the foundation's assumptions that they were "typically sharing a room with 95-year-old dementia patients." Berman said the foundation decided to limit the specialty houses to two because "We couldn't let our hearts run away with our wallets."

When I asked if anything has surprised him about the specialty houses at the Leonard Florence Center for Living since it opened, he said "Life expectancy is higher than we thought it would be, going in. For people with ALS, life there can be quite special." Although typically, this population might have a two to three year life expectancy, he said, the fact that doctors, nurse practitioners, and other clinicians stay on top of clinical issues, leads to fewer hospitalizations and a longer-term prognosis.

Last Comforts

If there is any example of what a life-changing difference living in a Green House can make, surely it is that of Steve Saling, who was diagnosed with ALS on Friday the 13th, 2006. He lives at the Leonard Florence Center of Living in the specialty house within the building for ALS patients. I met him virtually, via YouTube and email. Saling can't speak, but he communicates often and at length through a variety of media. Because his story is so remarkable, I want to share some of what he told me via email.

Saling met Barry Berman at an ALS symposium about six months after his diagnosis. "My symptoms were minor at the time but I knew what lay ahead of me and was proactively searching for a long term care solution so that I didn't end up stuck in a bed living in a chronic hospital for the rest of my life in what was and is still the norm," he said. "Barry was at the symposium with an idea of creating a specialized Green House to care for underserved disabilities like ALS but he had no idea if it were possible or how to go about it.

"We were each the perfect solution to each other's problems. He agreed to fully automate the ALS Residence and provide vent [ventilator] support. I agreed to use my architectural and universal accessibility experience along with my insight into ALS to design the perfect environment to live a productive life with ALS. We were a perfect partnership from that very first day."

He had temporarily moved back to his mother's house in Georgia in the Fall of 2007 and stayed there until Barry invited him to live in the organization's assisted living development the following Spring so he could be onsite to help

Nursing Home Transformation

in design and supervise construction of the Leonard Florence Center for Living. He moved into the newly constructed Green House in March 2010.

Since then, he's kept an active schedule. He often gives tours of his home and meets to discuss business issues. He typically works 40 hours a week, although not on a nine-to-five schedule. When no obligations are scheduled, he starts the day with breakfast in bed around 8:30, with a 15-minute tube feeding. It takes about an hour to get ready in the morning and situated in his wheelchair. He said he is usually "ready to roll" by 10:30. He spends the late morning and early afternoon taking care of online business and answering email, has lunch around 2 p.m. and then usually spends time in the living room.

"I am able to navigate my wheelchair independently with my head and with the PEAC automation [the Promixis Environment Automation Controller]. I don't have to call anyone," he said. "I am totally independent. I hang out with my housemates or go sit on the patio on a sunny day. Using PEAC, I can call the elevator and go downstairs and out of the building. In the summer, I have several nearby locations I like to go to, including a 20-acre, waterfront park just a five-minute walk away.

"In the evening, I often watch a movie with [a] buddy and housemate," he said. "I have music playing all day long. I usually go to bed between midnight and 1 a.m. It takes about 45 minutes to get me ready to sleep."

Remarkably, he has not been in bed for 24 hours straight since the day he was diagnosed.

Last Comforts

The experience of living in the Green House, he said, is "very much like family. Like family, we sometimes fight but we always make up. I'm frustrated that a few residents don't take advantage of the opportunities provided but it is their life. The staff gets to know us so well that I think they can read my mind. I often marvel at how well my needs are met, and try to keep that in mind when they're not."

Saling has been instrumental in advancing the technology that has enabled him to lead such a rich and purposeful life.

"In the beginning, I assumed there would be something available commercially," he explained, discussing the technology's evolution. "I quickly realized that wasn't the case. All of the operating hardware, like door openers, light switches, and power shades were readily available. The problem was there was no single interface to control them all. Barry and I had the help of an adaptive technology department of a major university but it became clear to me that we needed more help than a student class could provide.

"I struggled with the design of the project because I couldn't figure out how to provide power to all of the transmitters I would need on my wheelchair," he said. "I refused to have to be plugged in the wall. I began to realize I would need base computer to control everything and Eureka, the concept of PEAC was born."

Saling reached out to several automation companies and found one that understood his concept and was willing to customize. He and Barry Berman were still working with the university at that point. He convinced Berman they needed to turn away free help and hire a professional for several hundred thousand dollars. They signed a contract with Promixis and PEAC was developed.

"I use it all day every day. The freedom and independence it provides is beyond words. With it, I have complete control of my home theater. I can turn off, or dim the lights, lower the window shade, and watch TV or a movie. If it is warm, I can turn on a fan, the air conditioning, or both. I have full control of my HVAC. If the movie isn't streaming and I need someone to put a DVD in, I can use PEAC to call for assistance.

"I can open and close the door to my room and my house. I can call for the elevator and select the floor. All of this, I can do with my eyes using my computer. Because of the design, there is nothing to install on any wheelchair or on the computer. The only requirement is a wireless signal and a browser. It is the perfect solution. It is very intuitive to use and everyone is able to teach themselves. I frequently consult with Promixis to upgrade PEAC. I want it to become standard equipment where it's needed."

I wondered if he ever became blue, or discouraged, owing to the challenge of his illness. And, if he did, how did he cope?

He replied, "I get frustrated but I don't get depressed. Sometimes it kinda freaks me out because I realize how fucked up I must seem and that I should be more depressed. Depression just doesn't suit me."

Thinking about how Steve Saling lives his life, I couldn't help but think back to the time I'd spent with

Last Comforts

Bobby, whose struggle with ALS is described in Chapter 5. I wondered whether a nurturing home with able aides and advanced technology might have given him a chance to live out his days with some measure of comfort and perhaps real pleasure. There's no way of knowing, of course, but there is hope for others to follow.

❧❧

The nonprofit sector is in the forefront of culture change. In the U.S., roughly 15,500 nursing homes serve about 1.4 million residents at any given time. More than two-thirds of the homes are owned by for-profit companies. [5]

In contrast, "household" style nursing homes that embrace culture change are small-scale by their nature. These small-scale nursing homes represent, at this writing, only a small fraction of all long-term care residences. The most generous estimate I've heard is that households represent 5 to 10 percent of the total supply of nursing home beds. The question arises: Can these alternative long-term care models increase significantly over the next 20 years, enough so that we might come to expect this level of care as the norm?

The Centers for Medicare and Medicaid Services (CMS) helped clear any doubt about the legitimacy of household models in 2007, when it declared that no barriers prevent Green House developments from being qualified as nursing homes under federal regulations. However, financing household models for nursing homes is challenging. It was especially so during the recession of 2008–09 when financing for all commercial real estate was scarce.

Nursing Home Transformation

The federal government has provided the impetus for financing much of the long-term care industry. The U.S. Department of Housing and Urban Development (HUD), through its federal Housing Administration (FHA) Section 232 program, provides mortgage insurance on loans that cover housing for the frail elderly. This mortgage insurance provides lenders with protection against losses in the event that borrowers default on their mortgage loans. The program can be used to finance the purchase of a project, its refinancing, or new construction. HUD also backs major project rehabilitation. The federal government has provided incentives in certain instances via low-income housing tax credits and New Markets Tax Credits.

HUD has more than 2,900 active residential health care loans covering skilled nursing homes, assisted living facilities, and board and care facilities. A HUD spokesman could not pinpoint specific household-style developments for which it has insured mortgages, but he told me that there is no difference between household versus conventional nursing facilities in its underwriting approach. All such facilities are required to be state-licensed and meet the Medicare conditions of participation.

What About Financing?

Smaller developments have been successful in obtaining financing from local and regional banks, while larger developments have used tax-exempt bond financing, as was the case with Tockwotton. Nonprofit organizations have also tapped philanthropic organizations, private donors, and foundations and they have embarked on capital campaigns. Some have received land donated to them.

Hillcrest Health Services is a rare exception in the field because its household development in Papillion, Nebraska is a for-profit operation. Hillcrest President and CEO Jolene Roberts attended seminars about household developments and she studied the Green House model. She bought land for the proposed development in 2007.

"It was about the worst time to build," she said, "but we couldn't just sit on it." A delay in starting construction would mean losing the regulatory approval for the nursing home beds.

The Cottages at Hillcrest Country Estates consists of eight cottages of 13 elders, while a ninth was under construction when we spoke. Those eight cottages were built over four years starting in 2008. The only way she thought the concept would work in her market was to seek a conventional loan from a local bank where the company had done business for years. The fixed-rate loan, for 80 percent of the development cost, required a personal guarantee, something real estate developers usually shun wherever possible. For the 20 percent equity portion of the development cost, Roberts tapped investors with whom she'd previously done business. She expects the development to be financially stable and sustainable in 2018 when she hopes to take it to HUD.

Besides the economic challenges, Roberts said, "In Omaha, the concept was so foreign that people thought it was assisted living. People drove around asking 'where is the nursing home?' " Now the cottages are fully occupied, and have

Nursing Home Transformation

waiting lists.

Is it more expensive to build and operate a household model than it is to do a conventional nursing home? If so, does that threaten the potential financial sustainability of the household development? The answer is inconclusive.

Data for the costs of conventional nursing homes is plentiful because it is public information. Moreover, data can be gleaned from annual reports and SEC filings of large publicly held nursing home owners and operators. But understanding the financial health of household models is more problematic because there are still relatively few of them.

One person who has dived into the data for both is Ritchie Dickey, vice president of Lancaster Pollard, a financing and consulting firm whose clients include developers of both conventional skilled nursing facilities and household projects. Using data from the company's own household clients, Dickey set out, in 2010, to analyze the financial viability of building and operating these developments. Two years later, he revisited the topic, in a comparison between household developments and traditional nursing homes. By 2012, he found that while the cost of traditional nursing homes had varied little in those two years, the average cost for household projects had risen 10 percent.

Dickey focused on the average cost per bed for 20 proposed projects—both household and traditional. These costs included all financial expenses, but did not include the cost of land or site development, which can be considerable.

Traditional nursing beds ranged from 355 to 755 square feet per bed with costs ranging from $49,736 to $187,094. The median was $97,861.

Last Comforts

For a household with between 10 and 20 nursing beds, square footage per bed ranged from 500 to 1,400 square feet. Cost per bed ranged from $60,344 to $253,750. The median was $120,174.

Dickey said his company's clients showed that appropriate household models offer 16 to 20-unit modules (also called pods or neighborhoods) with a flexible staff. [6]

Martin Dickmann is formerly a financier with a private equity firm that owned nursing homes. Since 2008, he's been a partner and CFO at the consulting firm of Action Pact Development LLC. He said the sweet spot for financial viability for a household development is 20 to 22 beds per house. He estimates that between 60 and 80 units are needed for financial sustainability. (Action Pact provides development services, architectural design, operations, and management consulting services. Most of its clients are nonprofits.)

Contrary to the conventional wisdom, however, Dickmann said household developments do not necessarily cost more to construct than conventional nursing homes.

"People make bad decisions in any industry," he said. Mistakes might include picking materials and finishes that are too costly, or outfitting a 10-person household as extensively as one suited for 20, or buying land too expensively.

He offered this hypothetical comparison.

In a conventional 120-bed nursing home, you have a central kitchen, activity space, and between 65,000 and 75,000 square feet for 120 residents.

In a household development for 120 people, six 20-person households could comprise a total of 72,000

Nursing Home Transformation

square feet. Adding in six 300-square-foot kitchens (1,800 square feet) and common areas would result in the total square footage being comparable to a conventional development serving 120 people.

Construction costs are one factor. Operating costs are another. Is it more costly to operate a household model for elders than a nursing home? How is sufficient revenue generated to cover operating costs and mortgage payments?

Excluding interest payments, Dickmann said, staffing generally can represent a whopping 70 percent of a skilled nursing development's operating costs. Staff ratios are higher for 10-person households than for conventional skilled nursing homes. However, with more than 16 residents per house, households and conventional nursing homes could have similar staffing ratios. In Dickmann's hypothetical 120-bed household development with six 20-bed neighborhoods, additional staff would not be necessary, he said. Households could also achieve savings on food costs because there is less waste; on-demand cooking and leftovers could be managed.

In 2010, Ritchie Dickey questioned some of the assumptions that household developments were making in their financial projections, including margins of more than 20 percent. "That's not what you'd see," he said. Nursing costs also were projected at lower rates than he would expect to see. He is also concerned about household developments that are overbuilt, in terms of space, materials, and amenities. If they become financially troubled, that would cast a shadow for others in the field. Currently, he said, not enough information is widely available to make informed judgments.

Last Comforts

"In five years you could do a more rigorous analysis," he said.

Proponents of the household models argue that cost savings can be achieved because of the flatter management structure, lower staff turnover rates, and lower overall food costs. In terms of revenue, they say household models attract a higher percentage of private-pay residents (as compared to Medicare payments for short-term rehab or Medicaid payments for those who are without assets). If Medicaid is paying for more than half of the residents, it might be difficult to break even, but when the population is comprised of 50 percent private pay, that is sufficient for the household model to succeed, they say. Moreover, residents have been willing to travel longer distances and pay higher rates at household developments than they would for conventional nursing homes. A Midwest household development owner pegged a $100 per day difference between private pay and Medicaid reimbursement.

❧ ❧

Two developments underway—one in Connecticut and the other in Missouri—offer a glimpse of what the next iteration of household residences might look like. It's too early to tell whether they will be successful, but they bear watching because they offer a new element of enabling elders not only to live well, but also to remain connected with their communities.

The $60 million Liberty Project, in Liberty, Missouri is a proposed venture by Liberty Hospital, Healthy Living

Nursing Home Transformation

Centers of America, and Action Pact. Plans for the 22-acre development, near the Liberty Hospital campus, call for an integrated system centered on residents, easing transitions from one care setting to the next, and creating what its proponents call a true wellness center. Plans are for the project to be multi-generational and pedestrian-friendly, a development providing post-acute rehabilitation for Liberty Hospital patients, independent living, and skilled nursing.

The $42 million first phase of the development will comprise 60 suites of assisted living including memory-support skilled nursing; 60 suites in a separate building for what Tamera Evans, director of real estate at Liberty Hospital, called a short-term recovery hotel; and a health and fitness center. This phase is expected to be completed in Spring 2017. Plans for the second phase call for construction of 200 independent living units, along with retail, and medical office space.

Evans said that the goal is to keep seniors out of the hospital and integrated with the community. She acknowledged that "until people can touch it and see it," they might not understand how different the household model of care can be.

Integration with the community was also a guiding principle behind Jewish Senior Services' (JSS) Harry and Jeanette Weinberg Campus, which is slated to become the first household model in Connecticut. The campus will also include an 18,000-square-foot fitness center, an early childhood program, administrative offices, play spaces, library, gift shop, salon, theater, and restaurant. The intent is to host community events. The 372,000-square-foot development, on a nine-acre parcel in Bridgeport, is scheduled to open in Spring 2016 and is to include assisted-living apartments, short-term rehab households, and skilled nursing households, with private bedrooms and bathrooms.

Andrew Banoff, president of Jewish Senior Services, noted that seniors in nursing homes are often isolated. To counter that isolation, a JSS goal is to develop a multi-generational campus that includes adult day care. JSS also plans to replace its existing 360-bed nursing and rehabilitation facility with a household model nursing home, and to add assisted living apartments.

The project cost is nearly $100 million with 70 percent debt financing. Banoff believes it will be the largest household model nursing home in the country. He expects that up to 30 percent of the 14-bed skilled nursing households will be private pay. He also expects that operating costs will be comparable to conventional facilities.

Although Banoff has been approached by other organizations wanting to learn about the development, none are for-profit companies. "It's the nonprofit, mission-driven sector that has taken the lead" in household developments, he said.

New household models haven't yet made a major dent in the skilled nursing home world. With many of the nation's existing nursing homes 40 years or older, many are themselves aging and in need of more than simple facelifts. Operators who are embarking on physical makeovers might consider a philosophical and operational makeover to embrace culture change too.

Nursing Home Transformation

The Chelsea Jewish Foundation, for example, is renovating its traditional nursing facility (the Chelsea Jewish Nursing Home in Chelsea, Massachusetts) to incorporate the best of resident-centered design and care. The $16 million renovation of the 120-bed facility has torn out the building's central kitchen and nursing station and is transforming the residence. Inspired by the Green House model, its amenities, in 2016, are to include a day spa, café, chapel, fireplace, living rooms and lobby, and six 20-bed "homes" with kitchens but no private rooms.

Although the family-owned Windsor Healthcare Communities in New Jersey has not undertaken major physical redevelopment of its nine existing nursing homes, it has done something arguably more difficult. It is embracing organizational change.

After training with Eden Alternative, Vice President Batsheva Katz returned to Windsor with insights and new approaches to elder care.

"People come into this work because they have heart," she said when we met at Buckingham at Norwood, one of its Eden Alternative certified developments. "But they learn to separate that self out" when there are rigid policies, procedures, and regulations in place, as in a conventional nursing facility.

The better way, she said, is to empower the staff, recognize the worth of the universal care worker, flatten the hierarchy, provide consistent work assignments and create self-directed work teams. Why, for example, shouldn't a maintenance man be given the responsibility of giving an elder a shower, say, if he has developed a close rapport with that elder? (Katz said this was the case at one of Windsor's developments.)

Training is the key to culture change, Katz said, noting that the company spent $1 million on re-educating and training staff over six years. Rowena Sebastian, an occupational therapist, is Windsor's care trainer. After receiving training and certification at Eden Alternative, she teaches Windsor staff in small groups. The curriculum is not "one size fits all," she explained. It is tailored to individuals.

Windsor's tenth, and newest development is the Venetian Care and Rehabilitation Center in South Amboy, New Jersey. It opened in 2014. The three-story structure has 180 beds—60 beds for short-term, sub-acute care and 120 in skilled nursing. Each floor is equipped with two kitchens to serve the individual neighborhoods within the building.

Katz's brother, Windsor Vice President Joshua Jacobs remarked that "our financial structure is not remarkable" but differentiating it "is how we do things operationally, how we allocate the funds. The question is always, will this positively, or negatively impact the care of our elders?"

One of the big drivers behind Windsor's philosophy and operational approach is the imperative to prepare for aging baby boomers. The boomers want to live life to the fullest. They want choices, private rooms, quality customer service, and pleasant accommodations. "The leaders in the industry will rise to the challenge," Jacobs said.

More will rise to the challenge when consumers demand that they do so.

Chapter 11 Endnotes

1. Interview with Ray Rusin, chief, health facility regulation, Rhode Island Department of Health. The regulatory environment regarding skilled-nursing facilities varies from state to state. Rhode Island is one state that is committed to culture change. In 2009, after Rhode Island placed a moratorium on new nursing home beds, primarily to keep occupancy at 90 to 93 percent—the legislature exempted nursing home operators that developed a person-centered model. Rhode Island's nursing home regulations are here: webserver.rilin.state.ri.us/Statutes/title23/23-17/23-17-44.HTM

2. Improving Palliative and End-of-Life Care in Nursing Homes
www.pcori.org/research-results/2012/improving-palliative-and-end-life-care-nursing-homes

3. Koren's Long-Term Care Community Coalition acceptance speech
www.ltccc.org/news/documents/102214LTCCCMJKRemarksFINAL.pdf

4. The legend of the Shahbaz
www1.maine.gov/dhhs/reports/ltc-services/ShahbazLegend.pdf

5. "Overview of Nursing Facility Capacity, Financing and Ownership in the U.S. in 2011," Kaiser Family Foundation, June 2013. kff.org/medicaid/fact-sheet/overview-of-nursing-facility-capacity-financing-and-ownership-in-the-united-states-in-2011/

Chapter 11 Endnotes

6. On the financial viability of nursing home models:
www.lancasterpollard.com/NewsDetail/TCI-summer-
2010-sl-financial-viability-of-building-and-operating-house-
hold-projects. This 2010 study was based on 12 projects
proposed or built by clients of Lancaster Pollard. Here's the
2012 follow-up study.
www.lancasterpollard.com/NewsDetail/TCI-june-july-
2011-sl-household-projects-keys-for-success. 2012

12

Pathfinders in Coordinated Care

❝ Care should be 'and' instead of 'or.' ❞ —F. Amos Bailey, MD, palliative care pioneer, referring to the divide between curative treatment and comfort care.[1]

In the last few years of his life, my father was a frequent flyer. That is, he was in and out of hospitals for a variety of reasons. His hospital stays occurred in increasingly shorter intervals. He had a mild stroke, from which he recovered. He endured a stubborn urinary tract infection. In his remaining foot (in 1987, he'd had a below-the-knee amputation.), a deep sore developed in the big toe and that proved intractable despite many wound-care treatments in the hospital. All this occurred before the final five months of his life when he went from hospital to a post-acute rehab center, then back to the hospital. All of my father's ills were related to diabetes, but different specialists treated each ailment separately.

Last Comforts

Medical professionals use the term frequent flyer—though some just call it "the dwindles." The terms refer to people like my father who have frequent hospital stays and/or a pinball-like trajectory flinging them from hospital to a sub-acute rehab center, and then back home or to a nursing home, and then back to the hospital when they lurch into the next crisis. This pattern is common among the frail elderly who live with multiple chronic conditions. Like my father, their every hospital stay, and every transition from one care-setting to another, leaves them just a little weaker, maybe a little less mentally sharp or emotionally resilient and less able to engage in the everyday activities that give them pleasure.

Seventy-seven percent of Americans die from chronic illnesses, according to the National Center for Health Statistics. In the last two years of life, patients with chronic illnesses account for nearly one third of total Medicare spending—much of it for repeated hospitalizations. That's from research done by the Dartmouth Atlas of Health Care.

Forty-four percent of the two and a half million Americans who die each year do so while in hospice care. At the same time, aggressive care prior to hospice admission is rising. Intensive care admissions and repeat hospitalizations in the last 90 days of life have increased, as have the rates of transitions from one care setting to another in the last two weeks of life. In too many cases, hospice referrals come only in the last three days of life.

I spoke with Joan Teno, MD, associate director of the Center for Gerontology and Health Care Research at the Brown University School of Public Health. She is also lead author of an oft-cited study published in the Journal of the American Medical Association in 2013. [2]

Reporting on research comparing changes in end of life care for Medicare beneficiaries, the study looked at place of care, health care transitions, and site of death in 2000, 2005, and 2009.

"Once you get into acute care, that train is on the tracks and it's hard to derail it. We have created a [health care system] around the medical system, not around patients' needs," Dr. Teno said.

Care for patients who are checked in and out of hospitals and nursing homes near the end of their lives for cascading crises is typically uncoordinated. It is also not driven by goals of care developed through talks with a doctor, nurse practitioner, or social worker. Such treatment is also costly.

Worse, it is taxing, disruptive, and stressful for patients and their families. Every crisis can trigger worry, anxiety, and guilt, with family members asking, "Are we doing the right thing? How do we know the doctors are recommending the best possible care? Are we making the right decisions? Will there be a cascade of complications?"

Is there a way to obtain the kind of coordinated, interdisciplinary, and person-centered care that hospice provides without enrolling in hospice? The short answer is yes.

Some innovative health insurance providers and community organizations provide these services, as are leading retirement communities that offer continuing care at home. These programs are not new—some have been operating for as long as 20 years—and are gaining traction.

Last Comforts

Kaiser Permanente is one of the nation's largest managed-care companies. It has 9.5 million members in northern and southern California, as well as in seven other states and Washington, DC. Founded in 1945, KP has 38 hospitals and 17,425 physicians. Its physician medical groups provide care to its members. In 1996, its TriCentral region in southern California noticed that its hospice services were underused. Patients administered medically futile care often died in acute-care hospital beds or intensive care units. KP also found that nearly two-thirds of patients who died in the intensive care unit, and more than half of those who died in acute-care hospital beds, had a primary or secondary diagnosis of cancer, congestive heart failure, or chronic obstructive pulmonary disease (COPD).

For KP, that was a collective "aha!" moment. With assistance from the Partners in Care Foundation, KP established a pilot In-Home Palliative Care program in 1997 and then formalized it in 1998. The outpatient service, based in its Home Health Department, was designed to offer better care to dying patients and their families. This was a blended model of care, bridging traditional and hospice care. To be eligible, patients had to have cancer, congestive heart failure, or COPD. KP found these patients by asking their primary care physicians the simple question that palliative care pioneer Dr. Xavier Gomez-Batiste devised. That question has since become a beacon for palliative care practitioners.

It is this. "Would the physician be surprised if the patient died within a year's time?"

If patients had a life expectancy of one year, and had

230

one or more emergency department or hospital visits in the prior 12 months, they were eligible. Moreover, they did not have to forgo any curative treatments.

Thanks to its managed care structure and its ability to shift funds from hospital to home care, KP was able to implement and operate the program, said June Simmons, president and CEO of Partners in Care.

KP could not expand the innovative program without first measuring its effectiveness. A comparison study began in 1999 with patients divided into two groups. The control group consisted of home health patients who received usual care, that is, one nurse visit and access to the usual medical services. The palliative care group would have multiple home visits, access to an interdisciplinary team, and access to all of the usual medical services.

Palliative care physicians coordinated health care from a variety of providers, including the patients' primary care physicians and specialists. The core team included a physician, a nurse, and a social worker. All team members made home visits not only to provide medical care and support, but also to educate patients and their caregivers if needed. Support could include assistance with advance care planning so patients and their families could make informed decisions and choices about end-of-life care. Telephone support was available 24 hours a day, seven days a week.

The study revealed that members of the palliative care group were more satisfied with KP services than the control group was. Before they died, control group members had many more days either in emergency rooms or in the hospital than the palliative group did.

Dignity, comfort, pain, and symptom management, quality of care, and patient satisfaction were the program's hallmarks. Cost was not overlooked. The cost of caring for those in palliative care was 32.6 percent less than that of control group members.

In 2002 to 2004, with funding from the Garfield Memorial Fund, KP undertook further studies with 310 KP members in Colorado and Hawaii. A Partners in Care team conducted the random control trial and supported Richard Brumley, MD, and Kris Hillary, RN and nurse practitioner, who headed up home health and hospice in Tri Central at the time. They led the work, with Partners in Care collaborating with the measurement and project management team as well as preparing proposals, reports, and dealing with the institutional review board. The continued studies were as successful as the initial study. KP adopted the program as the standard of care throughout southern California and then rolled it out nationally.

"The model is so perfect for people. It kept people safe at home and reduced costs. It was very exciting and satisfying," said Partners in Care CEO June Simmons, who served on the Institute of Medicine committee that issued its Dying in America report in 2014.

The KP program for the palliative standard of care helped avoid, or it managed such symptoms as pain and nausea with much greater patient comfort and peace of mind than its earlier standard. Nor did patients have to wait for ambulances, go to the ER, or be treated by people who didn't know them. They avoided the risk of developing hospital-based infections, a possibility that becomes greater the longer a person remains in a hospital.

Other managed care and health insurance companies offer similar programs although they remain the exception rather than the rule. Simmons said, "It's so important to change the way we pay for things. We don't pay for home palliative care for the frail elderly population and we should."

Contemplating Mortality

To discuss the origins of Aetna's Compassionate Care program with its chief advocate, Dr. Randall Krakauer, Aetna's national medical director for Medicare, now retired, is to begin with a contemplation of mortality.

"We are a unique species; we don't accept mortality. Accepting one's mortality is a process, not an epiphany," Krakauer said.

Without that acceptance, he maintains, it is difficult to broach the important questions that we need to ask about how we want to live if serious illness befalls us. What kinds of treatments would we want? What treatments would we find intolerable? How do we want to live?

As he wrote in Frontiers Health Services Management in Spring 2011, "If our knowledge of our own mortality adds meaning to our lives, it should also empower us to choose some of the circumstances of our deaths."

He told me that after he'd graduated from medical school in 1972, it became clear in acute care settings that death was considered the enemy and all efforts were directed at making sure it didn't happen—even if it meant futile and aggressive treatment for patients. As recently as May 2014, he told a hearing of the Senate Special Committee on Aging, "In the last month of life among seniors, 80 percent of care is received in an acute care setting, often not medically reasonable or appropriate." [3]

Dr. Krakauer joined Aetna in 2004, recognizing that there remained a yawning gap between the kind of care patients wanted and needed and what they received. In light of the company's already robust case-management capability, he and the company leadership began thinking about how to change that. They wanted the primary focus to be on quality of care, not cost.

Aetna developed the Compassionate Care program for its insured to address patients with a life expectancy of 12 months. It enables them to have concurrent curative care along with palliative care. It offers unlimited inpatient hospice stays and does not limit spending on outpatient hospice stays. For family caregivers, the program offers 15 days of respite care plus bereavement services after a member's death.

A pilot program in January 2005 involved members representing 13 employers who used Aetna as their health insurance company. The pilot "succeeded beyond our most optimistic expectations," Dr. Krakauer said. The program boosted member satisfaction, dramatically increased hospice election, and it reduced use of acute care facilities.

The program has succeeded for Medicare Advantage members, too. Within this group, the hospice election rate

Pathfinders in Coordinated Care

has tripled to more than 80 percent. There was an 82 percent reduction in acute-care hospital days, an 88 percent reduction in intensive care days, and an 80 percent reduction in emergency room use. Aetna did not disclose its savings by going this route.

The company did this without incurring punishing administrative or training costs. It estimated the additional cost of attending to the needs of members with advanced illness at approximately $400 per nurse-case manager. While cost containment was not the primary goal, CMS calculated the savings in the Medicare Advantage group as more than $12,000 per participating member.

The nurse case-manager's role is the heart of the Compassionate Care Program, which serves approximately 7,700 individuals each year. Those individuals are either Aetna commercial members or Medicare Advantage members. Nurse case-managers coordinate care among patients' health care providers and provide culturally sensitive support. They discuss advance care planning choices and options with members and their families willing to talk about those issues. The nurse case-managers collaborate with social workers to identify needed resources, including home-delivered meals, financial advice, and transportation.

Those are the broad outlines. The sensitive work is done in the day-to-day contacts with members and their families.

Whenever one of her patients dies, Kathy Kendrek, a Registered Nurse and case manager with Aetna's Compassionate Care program, lights a candle on her desk and takes a few moments to honor that patient's memory. She calls the family to express her condolences and to thank them for allowing her the honor of working with them and their loved one. From time to time, she looks at the family photos, Christmas cards, notes, and letters she's collected since she began doing this work more than 10 years ago, saying "It reminds me why I'm doing this."

A hospice nurse at heart, Kendrek is that calm voice on the telephone helping patients or their caregivers when they are feeling scared and anxious, facing a crisis, or simply in need of assurance. Her goal is to make her clients feel valued, to "love them where they are."

What guides her, always, is a sense of how she herself would want to be treated.

For Kendrek, the important thing is to keep emphasizing that it is the member's choice as to how he or she wants to proceed. She tries to emphasize the benefits of palliative and hospice care, reminding them that studies have shown that people live longer if they're comfortable and not in pain. She emphasizes that they can always change their minds and opt for any procedures, such as CPR and feeding tubes.

"I will go so far as to read the definition of hospice and palliative care" to a member, she said. "Some people die without either. You never know what people are going to do."

Kendrek is one of five [registered? yes] nurses who became case managers when the program began in 2005. Each has a specialty and each has undergone special training in palliative care and cultural sensitivity. She has led "lunch and learn" sessions with the other nurses to keep improving their skills, and has served as a mentor in helping other nurses to have discussions about advanced illness with members and their families.

These nurses remember to take care of themselves, too.

Kendrek finds comfort in her faith and in talking with an Aetna social worker colleague. She tries to get enough sleep and exercise. "You can't be a wounded healer."

"What we're providing should be the standard of care," Dr. Krakauer said, pointing out that if these results had pertained to a drug or other innovative disease treatment, the medical community would likely be quick to embrace it. Embracing a process, though, is quite another matter.

Persuaded the Health Care System Must Change

Samira Beckwith dates her passion for caring for people with serious illness back some 40 years when she was diagnosed with Hodgkin's disease while a graduate student in social work at Ohio State University.

"I was supposed to be cured, but I was one of the five out of 100 who have a recurrence," she said. Besides being a lesson in how unpredictable the path of illness can be, her experience and her recovery gave her a lifelong sense of empathy with people who are ill. It also convinced her that the health care system had to change.

Beckwith is president and CEO of Hope HealthCare Services in Ft. Myers, Florida, a community organization serving

Last Comforts

8,000 people a year in three counties in southwest Florida. It began as Hope Hospice in 1983 serving 100 people a year.

"We want to help people make the transition from cure to care. That's always been my anchor," Beckwith said. Her commitment is to "walk with a person" along his or her final path. She does not like to use the words death or dying. She doesn't even like the phrase end-of-life. She prefers "final chapter."

How do they help that transition? "By providing the best care, the right care at the right time," she said.

But clearly, offering hospice care was not enough. There were so many people with chronic and serious illnesses who needed care, too. The challenge, she said, is that hospice has a 'box' drawn around it, circumscribed by regulations and reimbursement policies. So Beckwith and Hope started thinking about what supportive and caring services could be built around that box: providing help for people who were not hospice-eligible—and still be reimbursed for it.

Innovation rarely happens overnight. Beckwith started working on a Program of All-Inclusive Care for the Elderly (PACE) in 1999, but it took six years of work and making her case to state lawmakers before it was launched in 2006.

"One legislator once asked me, 'why are you working so hard on this?'" she recalled. Because people need it, she replied. Beckwith has since lent her expertise as a technical advisor to other organizations seeking to establish their own PACE programs.

Hope HealthCare Services has grown dramatically. Besides HopePACE, the organization also offers a community palliative care program, a children's hospice program, a Medicaid pediatric program for children who are not expected to live to be over 18, a Parkinson's disease support program, adult day centers, Community Care for the Elderly (CCE), specialized caregiver classes and grief programs. It employs 1,000 people and has 1,200 volunteers. Its annual operating budget is over $100 million.

PACE is a Medicare program—and a Medicaid state option—that provides community-based care and services to people 55 or older, who otherwise would need nursing home-level of care, but who can remain at home with assistance. The program uses the core skills of hospice, with an interdisciplinary team providing coordinated care focused on helping people achieve to their capability. For participants, PACE becomes their sole source of Medicare and Medicaid benefits. (For those who do not qualify for Medicaid, co-pays are required. The co-pays are equivalent to what Medicaid would pay for their services. At Hope HealthCare Services, 90 percent of participants are both Medicare- and Medicaid-eligible.)

What sets PACE apart from other forms of elder care is that it develops a plan of care for participants and covers all of the medical care they need, including medications and any visits with specialists, dentists, physical, or speech therapy. It also provides transportation to a community center several times a week, where the visits take place. At the centers, meals are available along with recreational and social activities. That combination simultaneously offers some respite time to caregivers. PACE also coordinates care at home, which may include help with meals and light housekeeping.

PACE was established in 1986, modeled on the work with elders that a Chinatown-based community group, now known as On Lok Lifeways, had done in San Francisco beginning in 1973. Beckwith started working on a Program of All-Inclusive Care for the Elderly (PACE) in 1999, but it took six years of work and making her case to state lawmakers before it was launched in 2006.

On Lok Lifeways began with a senior-day health-care center and has since grown to become a complete medical- and health-related services program. A turning point came in 1983, when it obtained waivers from Medicare and Medicaid to test a new financing method for long-term care: a form of risk-based capitation. That is, in exchange for fixed monthly payments from Medicare and Medicaid for each enrollee, On Lok was responsible for delivering a full range of health care services, including hospital and nursing home care—bearing the full financial risk. A permanent Medicare and Medicaid waiver followed in 1986.

In 1986, CMS, the Robert Wood Johnson Foundation, and the John A. Hartford Foundation provided On Lok with funds to replicate its model at 10 additional sites. The success of these demonstration projects led to its establishment as a permanent program within Medicare. In the federal Balanced Budget Act of 1997, PACE became a permanent provider type under Medicare, and states gained the option of paying a capitation rate for PACE services under Medicaid.

According to the National PACE Association, which was formed in 1994 with 11 PACE organizations operating in nine states, there are now 107 programs in 31 states. (In Pennsylvania, the program is known as Living Independence for the Elderly, or LIFE). Nearly half of PACE participants have dementia, but 90 percent can live in the community. (To find out if there is a PACE program in your area, visit www. pace4you.org.)

The association reports that its "typical" participant is an 80-year-old woman living with eight medical conditions and challenges in three activities of daily living. (There are six basic activities of daily living: eating, bathing, dressing, toileting, transferring—being able to move from one place to another—and continence.)

In its report in Evidence Matters, the U.S. Department of Housing and Urban Development noted: "In addition to better clinical outcomes through shorter hospital stays, lower mortality rates, and better self-reported health and quality of life, costs for PACE enrollees are estimated to be 16 to 38 percent lower than Medicare fee-for-service costs for the elderly population and 5 to 15 percent lower than costs for comparable Medicaid beneficiaries." [4]

Continuing Care at Home

For people of means who want coordinated health care and assistance when they need it, but don't wish to move to an assisted living or continuing care development, continuing care at home is a growing alternative. The caveat: you cannot wait until a crisis occurs; you must be healthy and independent when you sign on. It is not cheap. There is typically an entrance fee (which may or may not be refundable), plus a monthly fee. Fees can vary widely, depending on your age when you sign on, and what level of services you want. Some offer portability—that is, if you are connected to a company in one state, but move to another state, you will still be covered.

Typically, continuing care at home offers a package of services aimed at supporting you medically, spiritually and socially. It can be your advocate. It includes an annual physical and provides care coordination, home inspections, an emergency response system, homemaker and personal care services (live-in, if needed), meals, home nursing, and transportation. It can also provide social, recreational, and educational activities, or an adult day program, at its own campus. It can refer you to home maintenance, lawn care, and housekeeping services, if you need those too. Like Aetna's Compassionate Care program, care coordinators are the heart of continuing care at home services.

Kendal at Home in Westlake, Ohio, is an affiliate of the Kendal Corp., which comprises not-for-profit retirement communities, programs, and services founded on the principles of the Religious Society of Friends (Quakers). Lynne Giacobbe, executive director of Kendal at Home, described how she had been impressed watching the first hospice program being developed in her community when she was a teen. Her mother had had been the first head nurse in the cancer unit of a local hospital.

"This program, in so many ways, mirrors what hospice does," she said. "It's based on the same philosophy." The care coordinator's role is critical. As one example, Giacobbe told me about a care coordinator who helped ease a member's passing and provided comfort for the member's daughter at the same time. The member had end-stage lung disease and as it progressed, she was transferred to an inpatient hospice where she rallied but then worsened. The daughter did not live nearby and her main fear was that her mother would die alone. The care coordinator had gotten to know the member very well, and had sensed that the woman needed the daughter to assure her that the daughter would be okay after the woman died. At the end, the care coordinator arranged for the two to talk by phone, keeping it on speaker. The daughter did provide assurance to her mother, saying it was okay to let go. They stayed connected, quietly, as the mother's breathing calmed and she died peacefully.

Giacobbe, whose background had been in victim services, was hired by Kendal at Home in 2003. A year later, the program was launched to serve 10 counties in northern Ohio by holding its first seminar for prospective members. The program now covers 250 members. For those under 75, there is a one-time fee of under $50,000 plus a monthly fee, on average, of $650 (depending on the level of coverage, co-pay, and refundable options).

The program contracts for most of the care it provides. Giacobbe said it spends a million dollars in private duty care every year.

What has surprised her is that some adult children of members seem like they would be involved in their parents' care, but aren't, although there are many who are. Challenging, too, is that many of the adult children do not live in northern Ohio. An important part of the care coordinator's responsibilities is to communicate with the adult children.

Longwood at Home is a service of Presbyterian SeniorCare, a non-profit, faith-based network of living and care options, serving older adults in 10 counties in western Pennsylvania. Director Joan Krueger explained that Longwood at Home got its approval from the state Department of Insurance in late 2002 and began actively marketing the program a year later. It has close to 300 members.

"Our members tend to be fiercely independent and they want to be in a multi-generational community and remain involved with their community," she said, noting that they have, in effect, two generations of members: the youngest member is 62 and the oldest is 102. She expects that fewer than five percent of these members will ultimately move to a continuing care retirement community permanently.

The staff is small: four care coordinators with backgrounds in social work. Typical of the kind of sensitivity the care coordinators bring to their role, she explained, involved the case of a man who was in the early stages of dementia. The organization where he had been a volunteer asked him to resign, but the care coordinator was able to find another organization where he was welcome and could maintain a sense of purpose. The coordinator also found him an aide who shared his avid interest in the outdoors and who hikes with him regularly.

There are six different plans available at Longwood at Home. They range widely from an initial payment of $5,000 for 60-year-olds who want home care only, to more than $160,000 for those 88 or older, 90 percent of which is refundable. Monthly fees vary, too; they are higher if the member wants the option of facility-based coverage. For those who have been members for more than a year, coverage is portable.

Krueger see significant growth for Longwood at Home in the next five years, but she recognizes that particularly as boomers age, the continuing care at home business is going to have to change and become more flexible. In 2014, a survey of 1,000 people by Natixis Global Asset Management revealed that one third of boomers have saved less than $50,000. The average savings among boomers was under $275,000—which could dampen prospective members' enthusiasm for paying large entrance fees. [5]

Scott E. Townsley, principal at the certified public accounting and consulting firm CliftonLarsonAllen, which has worked with many senior housing and skilled nursing companies, told me that there has not been dramatic growth in the field and further, that he expects that in the next five years there will be some failures in the business. Those are likely to take place among organizations that shouldn't have been in the business in the first place, or whose management didn't expect to find the field as complex as it is.

Washington Begins to Notice

The potential benefits of coordinated care have not gone unnoticed in Washington, DC. It does often seem as if the many hours devoted to crafting Medicare regulations and payment policies only nibble around the edges of the critical issues, with a focus on rooting out potential fraud and abuse, tweaking regulations to address drug reimbursements here, or tightening hospice eligibility there—all in an effort to keep a lid on taxpayer expenditures.

Should there be more frequent inspections of hospices? Should the per-diem hospice reimbursement rate be paid differently to reflect higher use of hospice resources when a person first comes to hospice care and then when it rises again, in the last several days before death? What should be considered primary diagnoses, for eligibility, and to what extent must continuing decline occur? These are questions that have taken up much time in Washington. The impact of amended rules ripples out widely to affected organizations. Systemic change often seems incremental, small-bore, and frankly not attuned to addressing the essential question of how we can make people's lives just a little better toward the end.

But the idea of offering coordinated care, and non-medical support, to people who are frail and ill does have its champions. Three of the Center for Medicare and Medicaid Innovation (CMMI) demonstration projects—mandated by the Affordable Care Act—are worth noting: the Medicare Care Choices pilot project; Independence at Home; and the Community Based Care Transitions Program.

Medicare's Care Choices pilot project, announced in 2014, allows certain hospice patients—Medicare beneficiaries and those who are dually eligible for Medicare and Medicaid—to elect hospice care without having to give up curative treatments.

Pathfinders in Coordinated Care

The pilot project focuses on those who have advanced cancers, chronic obstructive pulmonary disease (COPD), congestive heart failure, or HIV/AIDS. Originally, CMS was going to pick at least 30 rural and urban Medicare-certified and enrolled hospices to participate. It expected to enroll 30,000 beneficiaries over a three-year period. But because there was so much interest in the pilot, CMS expanded the model to more than 140 Medicare-certified hospices and extended the duration of the model from three to five years. This is expected to enroll as many as 150,000 eligible Medicare beneficiaries

In announcing the project, former Senate Finance Committee Chairman Ron Wyden (D-OR), who sponsored the provision authorizing the program, said, "This initiative represents a fundamental change in the way health care is delivered. Patients and their families should have every choice available to them when faced with life-threatening illness. Allowing Medicare coverage to continue while under hospice care means that patients no longer have to make a false choice between hospice and curative care."

CMS will pay a $400 fee per beneficiary per month to participating hospices for services. This is less than what it typically pays per person for conventional hospice care. Providers and suppliers furnishing curative services to beneficiaries participating in the the Medicare Care Choices Model program will be able to continue to bill Medicare as they ordinarily would.

After the pilot is done, there will ideally be useful evidence about whether concurrent care encourages more people

Last Comforts

to sign on to hospice, improves their quality of life, and results in lower Medicare costs. [6]

Most professionals I spoke to since the project was announced are eager to watch how it progresses. They hope it will lead to a change in how end-of-life care is reimbursed, although some remained skeptical not only because it limits the kinds of diagnoses that would be covered but also because the reimbursement rates are considered too paltry to attract many organizations that would otherwise have sought participation. Others were concerned about a possible negative effect if the results yield no significant cost savings.

Like PACE programs, the Independence at Home (IAH) Demonstration is intended to encourage the delivery of high-quality primary care in a home setting, using an interdisciplinary team approach to coordinate care. In all, there were 17 participating practices serving more than 8,400 Medicare beneficiaries.

In its first performance year, CMS announced that the demonstration did show higher quality care (including fewer hospital readmissions within 30 days) and lower Medicare expenditures. The demonstration saved $25 million, an average of $3,070 per beneficiary.

Beneficiaries were selected to participate if they had two or more chronic conditions; had original, fee-for-service (FFS) Medicare coverage; needed assistance with two or more activities of daily living; had a non-elective hospital admission within the previous 12 months; and had received acute or subacute rehabilitation services in the prior 12 months. In the demonstration, beneficiaries with conditions such as diabetes,

Pathfinders in Coordinated Care

high blood pressure, asthma, pneumonia, or urinary tract infections used fewer inpatient hospital and emergency services.

With these results, not surprisingly, advocates for elder health care are calling for the Independence at Home (IAH) Demonstration to become a chronic care coordination benefit under Medicare.

The Centers for Medicare and Medicaid (CMS) launched the Community-Based Care Transitions Program (CCTP) in 2012, with the goal of improving transitions of Medicare beneficiaries from inpatient hospitals to home or other care settings. Community-based organizations (CBOs) use care-transition services to improve quality of patient care, which, in turn, helps to reduce hospital readmissions, and achieves cost savings for Medicare. The CBOs are paid an all-inclusive rate per eligible discharge based on the cost-of-care transition services for the patient and implementing the systemic changes made by the hospital. By mid-June 2013, CCTP agreements were awarded to 101 community-based organizations and 461 acute-care hospitals that partnered with the community-based organizations. The program is funded for five years.

Perhaps this pilot project will find what Mt. Sinai Health System in New York City already has. Mt. Sinai found that when social workers had the opportunity to go into the community and learn about nonmedical reasons behind frequent emergency room and hospital use, the system addressed them, with the result that 30-day hospital readmissions dropped dramatically. What were some of those issues? Overwhelmed family caregivers, or lack of family support, unsafe housing, high levels of family violence and trauma, poor literacy, language barriers and untreated mental illness. [7]

"The people we're trying to serve aren't interested in a good death; they're interested in a good life," and for elders, independence is valued more highly than longevity, Dr. Diane E. Meier told attendees at Atlantic Health Systems' annual palliative care symposium held at Overlook Hospital in Summit, New Jersey in May 2014. Dr. Meier is director of the Center to Advance Palliative Care, the national organization devoted to educating the public about, and increasing the number and quality of palliative care programs in the United States. She is also a professor of geriatrics and palliative medicine at Mount Sinai School of Medicine in New York City.

She shared an anecdote with her audience (mostly residents, nurses, and chaplains) about Mr. and Mrs. B, both in their eighties, he more frail than she. Mt. Sinai's palliative care team had been called to consult on the case of Mr. B because he was "abusing the emergency system," she explained. Why was that? Because when a crisis happens after normal business hours, as most of us have found out at some point, a recorded message in the physician's office instructs us to call 911 in an emergency. That's what they did.

With coordinated care through the palliative care team, Mr. and Mrs. B now can call for assistance 24/7. They receive Meals on Wheels, mainly to help Mrs. B in her caregiver role. The team also arranged for their local church to have volunteers visit them three times a week. With these changes, the couple did not return to the emergency room once in 18 months.

Pathfinders in Coordinated Care

"Palliative care is about improving quality of life. A side effect is that it reduces the need for acute-care emergency services," she said.

But Medicare currently does not pay for the kinds of help that would enable the frail or seriously ill to live a good life as they themselves would define it. Among its recommendations on policy and payment systems, the Institute of Medicine report on Dying in America there was this.

"Federal, state, and private insurance and health care delivery programs should integrate the financing of medical and social services to support the provision of quality care consistent with the values, goals, and informed preferences of people with advanced serious illness nearing the end of life. To the extent that additional legislation is necessary to implement this recommendation, the administration should seek and Congress should enact such legislation."

Easier said than done. But as Dr. Meier told symposium attendees, "The more we go away from fee-for-service, the closer we'll get to funding for personal care."

Mid-Life Crisis for Hospice

It seems to me that at 40-something, hospice in the U.S. is having its mid-life crisis. Maybe it is time to start from scratch and design benefits based on people's needs, not on their prognoses, as Dr. F. Amos Bailey suggested. He led open-access palliative and hospice care programs in Alabama and in the Veterans Administration.

I think about Alice whose story is told in Chapter 4.

Last Comforts

I used to visit her in a nursing home. Frail, demented and in her nineties, she spent her days in bed, isolated, sleeping when she wasn't awake, and often hallucinating. Her diagnosis was "debility" before that term was eliminated as a primary diagnosis for hospice coverage. She became a "live discharge"— not because she had achieved a miraculous recovery, but because she was deemed to have become stable and therefore, no longer eligible for hospice services.

Was she suddenly less in need of the extra compassionate care that hospice offered her? I don't think so. If she was like others discharged from hospice, she might have felt abandoned, confused, and fearful. But hospices are under increasing pressure—as is CMS, for that matter—to question hospice care particularly for nursing home residents who tend to stay in hospice care longer than people who remain in their own homes. One reason for this is that, especially with dementia, decline often does not follow a straight-line pattern. As one hospice administrator told me, the path is more like a saw-tooth.

There are other reasons why nursing home residents tend to stay in hospice care longer. Hospice has strayed far from its historical roots. The preponderance of hospices now are for-profit operations, and more than a few have been found to put profits ahead of compassionate care. Because hospice is paid a per-diem rate of about $150, it is more profitable to sign up people who will stay in hospice care longer. Those people tend to be nursing home residents.

Reimbursement is higher, too, for people who must receive general inpatient care. The latter involves figuring out a regimen of medications to address pain, or continuous care when the person's needs are complex.

Because hospice covers all care related to a person's primary diagnosis, that might include, say, palliative radiation or chemotherapy to shrink a tumor for the sake of comfort. Those treatments are costly. The danger is that people will be discharged from hospice care before a bottom-line-oriented hospice organization becomes responsible for such treatments.

It is a system that virtually invites gaming by those with ill intent. It has led to fraud, abuse, and waste by bad actors in the system. It has led to cases of insufficient care; recruiting people to sign up for hospice when they were not dying—largely from nursing homes; premature discharges from hospice to avoid costly palliative treatments, among other egregious practices. All this has forced CMS and hospices to take a closer look at their clients, the length of service, and type of care provided.

What should be the way forward? Instead of nibbling around the edges of hospice care policy and payment, let's design a system that can support the most vulnerable among us. Let's recognize that nonmedical support is critically important. Let's give broader access for the ill and their caregivers to professionals who can coordinate care and counsel them by phone, any time of day or night. Let's weed out the bad actors in the business. And finally, let's not punish people for failing to die on time.

Chapter 12 Endnotes

1. ER interview with F. Amos Bailey, MD, December 3, 2014.

2. Joan M. Teno, MD, MS. *et al.* "Change in End-of-Life Care for Medicare Beneficiaries: Site of Death, Place of Care, and Health Care Transitions in 2000, 2005, and 2009." *JAMA.* 2013. 309(5):470–77. doi:10.1001/jama.2012.207624. Feb. 2013

3. Dr. Krakauer testified about the Compassionate Care program at a hearing May 21, 2014 of the Senate Special Committee on Aging.
www.aging.senate.gov/hearings/roundtable-continuing-the-conversation_the-role-of-health-care-providers-in-advance-care-planning

4. *Evidence Matters*, "Measuring the Costs and Savings of Aging in Place." Fall 2013. Evidence Matters, a HUD publication www.huduser.org/portal/periodicals/em/fall13/highlight2.html

5. More troubling news about baby boomers' savings: In April 2015, the Insured Retirement Institute reported that 6 in 10 Americans, aged 52 to 68, approaching retirement or already retired, had savings while four in 10 reported no savings. Twenty percent have $250,000 or more saved. Nearly 6 in 10 have made no preparations in the event they experience cognitive issues. The survey was of 803 Americans.

Chapter 12 Endnotes

The Institute has been conducting these surveys since 2011. "Boomers' Confidence in Secure Retirement Sinks to Five-Year Low," April 13, 2015: www.irionline.org/resources/resources-detail-view/boomer-2015

6. More information about the Medicare Care Choices pilot project is at innovation.cms.gov/initiatives/Medicare-Care-Choices/.

7. http://www.ehcca.com/presentations/predmodel6/kalman_1.pdf7.

13

A Better Future and A Call to Action

"Future policymakers must…recognize the urgent need to address certain issues that have long been considered extremely difficult both politically and legislatively. They include financing and improving the quality of long-term care; embracing innovative approaches to palliative care and confronting issues around the end of life… If we are to achieve meaningful success, it will take more than good policy and superior technology. It will also take enlightened leadership."—Thomas Daschle, writing about "Fifty Years In, Medicare Has Transformed Health Care. What's In Store For The Next Fifty?" in Health Affairs. [1]

Last Comforts

You might have heard about the highlights of the 1964 World's Fair in Flushing Meadows in New York City. "Peace Through Understanding" was its optimistic theme. Progress both cultural and technological was its promise. General Motors had one of the more popular pavilions, offering its elaborate "Futurama" vision: undersea communities; colonies on the moon; cars whisked along efficiently via moving highways. More than 50 years later, we see how that turned out. Would anyone have predicted the demise and rebirth of mighty General Motors itself?

Predicting the future can be dicey. Still, let's fast forward to 2035. What do you imagine? Better treatments, maybe even cures found even for fatal cancers? Personalized medicine and treatment based on your DNA? Discovery of a way to prevent dementia, or to treat it effectively if it can't be prevented? Technology and robotics capable of replacing lost limbs or organs? Enabling physicians, care coordinators, or long-distance caregivers to monitor our health remotely and in real time, and to respond quickly if worrisome changes occur?

These may all be within the realm of possibility—and what we can hope for. Nevertheless, there still won't be a cure for mortality. There will still be a need to help frail elders not only with the basics of what they need to live with a modicum of dignity, but also with the human touch of companionship that helps make life worth continuing to live.

As described in these pages, the seeds for a better future for care through the close of life have been planted.

A Better Future and A Call to Action

Here are my nominations for the Top 20 elements in an ideal world. It is a future where:

1. As patients, our voices are heard and honored when we tell our team of health care professionals what matters most to us.

2. High quality care is available to all, regardless of race, ethnicity, economic status, sexual, or gender orientation.

3. We will be able to talk with a palliative care team shortly after receiving a diagnosis of serious illness. That conversation won't have to wait until we are in mid-crisis.

4. Palliative care is available wherever we need it, not just in the hospital, but at home, in the community, or in an assisted living, continuing care, or skilled nursing facility. It is available not just in large urban centers, but in suburbs, and in rural communities where accessing such care has been challenging.

5. Our health care team communicates with one another, shares information about us and shares the same goals for us; our records and our advance-care plans travel with us, to whichever care setting we need.

6. The burden of being "quarterback," or chief coordinator of communication and information, does not fall on the responsibility-laden shoulders of our caregivers.

7. Our physicians, nurses, and direct care workers understand the challenges of caring for elder patients—even if they are not specialists in geriatrics or palliative care.

8. A new generation of doctors and nurses is accustomed to working together in teams to care for their patients.

Last Comforts

This generation views palliative care not as the red-headed stepchild of the medical profession but rather as a central component of patient-centered care, at the heart of why they wanted to join the medical profession to begin with.

9. Communities are able to identify those most in need of the kind of coordinated, nonmedical social support that will enable people to live as well as possible in the community, without repeated emergency room visits and hospitalizations.

10. If we need to be hospitalized and must stay in post-acute rehabilitation or in a skilled nursing facility afterward, important information about our care and our own values will not fall between the cracks in making transitions from one setting to another.

11. If we need long-term care for complex medical or cognitive issues, we have a choice of many skilled facilities adhering to the principles of culture change and patient-centered care so we will not feel isolated and warehoused.

12. People of color and LGBT elders will no longer fear being abused, neglected, or otherwise mistreated and discriminated against in long-term care settings.

13. Operators of long-term care facilities train and empower certified nursing assistants (CNAs), home health aides, and personal care aides and pay them a living wage to reflect their advancing skills.

14. A new form of reimbursement will have been crafted to adequately reimburse medical practitioners for high-quality care for nursing home residents at the end of their lives, without the extra overlay of hospice agency involvement

A Better Future and A Call to Action

(thus eliminating one major opportunity for spurious practices by the bad actors in the field).

15. Elders with dementia are cared for by skilled and well-trained staff who understand how to balance stimulation and relaxation, to help elders have as good a day as possible, every day.

16. Elders who are alone, without children, family or friends to support them—the "unbefriended," as some advocates call it—will have a supportive community to care for them.

17. At least one major politician or celebrity will have made news by ceremoniously filling out an advance care directive and explaining its importance to the public.

18. Subsequently, most older adults will have made their wishes and preferences known, and will have designated a health care proxy to speak for them if they can't speak for themselves.

19. The subjects of illness and end-of-life issues will have become common in popular culture, books, TV, movies, and digital media that explore in dramatic, comedic, and combinations of both, the myriad aspects of human drama and spirit at work at the close of life.

And at long last...

20. The wall between what had been considered "curative" treatment and comfort care will be permanently demolished, having yielded to a health-care policy and payment system that embraces both approaches concurrently without costing taxpayers more than the current system that is fragmented, costly, often dysfunctional, and unsustainable.

261

Last Comforts

Incremental Progress

We have a long way to go to get to this version of our future. Thankfully, legions of people in the public, academic, philanthropic, and private sectors are working to achieve progress. It is painstaking work, meticulous and incremental, but it is progress.

Going forward, we're going to hear a lot about measuring quality of care. What should good palliative and end-of-life care look like? The American Academy of Hospice and Palliative Medicine (AAHPM) and the Hospice and Palliative Nurses Association (HPNA) have tackled this question, working with hundreds of health care professionals before jointly devising their top ten "Measuring What Matters" quality indicators for treating patients with serious or life-threatening illness. (The ten are outlined in Chapter 14.) These are recommendations only, an excellent start.

Joseph Rotella, MD, chief medical officer of the AAHPM, told me "The way we measure quality needs to be more patient-centered." In 5 or 10 years, he fully expects that the science of quality measurement will develop rapidly, leading to improved patient care.

Palliative care, he said, should address patients' needs wherever they are and should include family and spiritual support and help with practical problems. "With the right care at the right time, people do better and feel better."

Some institutions have begun to define quality for themselves. At the Providence Institute for Human Caring, part of Providence Health and Services in southern Cali-

A Better Future and A Call to Action

fornia, Ira Byock, MD, palliative care pioneer and now the institute's chief medical officer, discussed its major priority, currently, to "change internal expectations and define what quality looks like, making sure that care plans reflect good faith efforts to value patients' goals, values, and preferences." More specifically, it will define what quality looks like to cardiac patients, Alzheimer's patients, cancer patients, patients in the ICU, and primary care for adults of Medicare age.

These quality expectations will be translated into practice settings, education and system design and outcome measurement, he said. The linchpin in all of this? The quality of conversations, Dr. Byock said.

Providence is also working on charting templates for conversations about goals of care.

The Centers for Medicare and Medicaid Services has itself developed a data collection tool for use in scoring quality of care in hospices based on seven measures of quality. CMS has also developed a post-death family caregiver survey to get a better handle on patient and family experiences with hospice care. Data submission by hospices was slated to begin, quarterly, in August 2015. The seven quality measures are:

1. Patients, treated with an opioid, who are given a bowel regimen: The percentage of vulnerable adults (including hospice patients) treated with an opioid that are offered/ prescribed a bowel regimen or documentation why this was not needed.

2. Pain Screening: The percentage of hospice or palliative care patients who were screened for pain during the hospice admission evaluation / palliative care initial encounter.

3. Pain Assessment: The percentage of hospice or palliative care patients who screened positive for pain and who received a clinical assessment of pain within 24 hours of screening.

4. Dyspnea Screening: The percentage of hospice or palliative care patients who were screened for dyspnea during the hospice admission evaluation / palliative care initial encounter. (Dyspnea is difficult or labored breathing; shortness of breath.)

5. Dyspnea Treatment: The percentage of patients who screened positive for dyspnea who received treatment within 24 hours of screening.

6. Treatment Preferences: The percentage of patients with chart documentation of preferences for life-sustaining treatments.

7. Beliefs/Values Addressed (if desired by the patient): The percentage of hospice patients with documentation of a discussion of spiritual/religious concerns, or documentation that the patient/caregiver/family did not want to discuss. [2]

The Role of Technology

We are also going to hear a lot more in the years ahead about the role of technology. No one has yet come up with a disruptive palliative and end-of-life care equivalent of Uber or Airbnb, but many start-ups are trying.

The enormity of the baby boom cohort will certainly give rise to new, tech-driven opportunities to cater to us in our old age. The mission of an organization called Ag-

A Better Future and A Call to Action

ing2.0® is to accelerate innovation to improve the lives of older adults around the world. Over the past few years, Aging2.0 has hosted more than 100 events in 22 cities across nine countries, attracting innovators, entrepreneurs, technologists, designers, investors, and long-term care providers.

Not coincidentally, Aging2.0 also uses its platform to find likely businesses to invest in. It is part of Generator Ventures, launched in May 2014 in conjunction with Formation Capital, a $6 billion private equity firm focused on seniors' housing and care, post-acute, and health-care real estate investments. Generator Ventures provides capital and access to long-term care organizations and distribution channels. Aging2.0's Academy program is tied closely to Generator Ventures. Participation in the Academy program is the first step on the road to possible investment by Generator Ventures.

Other venture capital firms are dipping their toes into what Scott Collins, CEO of Link-age and others in the field call the "longevity economy." Link-age comprises three companies, all focused on the aging population. One of the three is Link-age Ventures, an investor that has partnered with Ziegler, a leading investment banker in the senior living business. In July 2014, Ziegler Link-age Longevity Funds closed on a $26.6 million fund and within a year had invested in several companies.

The fund's investors include 70 nonprofit companies with a network of 600 senior living communities in the U.S. The investors, Collins told me, are naturally keen to achieve a good economic return, but they are also very interested

265

in ways to incorporate technological innovations into their business models. He pointed out that hotels have traditionally been at the cutting edge of technology. Eventually hotel innovations are adapted by hospitals and later, by long-term care operators. The investors' goal, he said, is to find ways to shorten the time in that cycle.

The field is evolving rapidly. Collins said his company's focus is to find companies using technology to better manage chronic diseases; to create more connectivity through the care continuum (from the hospital to post-acute care to long-term facilities); to measure quality and apply metrics to improve patients' quality of life; to achieve better outcomes by encouraging patients to stick to their drug regimens; to avoid adverse drug reactions; and to give the right drugs at the right doses; and to enhance social connectivity—particularly for those who are not tech-savvy.

A Focus on Community

It takes a village to raise a child, as the saying goes. As the decade rolls on, expect to hear more about how it will take a village to care for our elders, too. Many of the solutions to be crafted will be intensely local in nature.

Joanne Lynn, MD, is one of the fiercest advocates for care for the frail elderly. One of the first hospice doctors in the country, she is now head of the Center for Elder Care and Advanced Illness (CECAI), chartered in 2011 by the nonprofit Altarum Institute.

"We've set ourselves up for a crisis. Most people will

A Better Future and A Call to Action

have a substantial period of disability," she said. "People have enough to live on until they get sick." At the same time, Medicare is riddled with wasteful policies and services such as paying for futile tests, procedures, and treatments. "We have to make it possible to spend public money more prudently." That means funding supportive services.

CECAI proposes what it calls the MediCaring Accountable Care Community initiative, which is designed to provide higher quality care for frail elderly Medicare beneficiaries at a lower per capita cost than is currently the case. The savings generated would help fund long-term, community-based services and supports, using a modified Accountable Care Organization (ACO) known as an Accountable Care Community (ACC). A community board would monitor the quality and supply of services.

Dr. Lynn is perplexed that MediCaring seems to be the only such detailed proposal for comprehensive services introduced. "There should be many more," she said.

In the meantime, absent a big increase in funding for services provided under the Older Americans Act (OAA), the number of low-income elders in need of services (through its Title III grants) such as meals, transportation, and home-based services is likely to soar.

The OAA, signed into law in 1965, was designed to help elders remain in their homes and communities. Much of the funding for Meals on Wheels, for example, which serves 2.5 million elders annually, is through Title III grants. A comparative note: it costs less to provide an elder with Meals on Wheels for a year than it costs to spend one day in the hospital or six days in a nursing home, according to Meals on Wheels America. [3]

But the OAA does not meet the current need, let alone future needs. A recent Government Accountability Office study of "The Older Americans Act and Unmet Needs" noted that while funding to states for Title III programs has decreased since 2009, the number of older adults increased from 55.5 million to 62.9 million in 2013. It estimated that 90 percent of low-income adults who likely need meal services do not receive them. [4]

According to the Altarum Institute, funding for the OAA has increased less than five percent over ten years. At this writing, Congress has not reauthorized the OAA, much less proposed increased funding.

Until programs such as MediCaring, or Independence at Home (discussed in Chapter 12) become a reality, what are frail elders to do? Christine Ritchie, MD, is a board certified geriatrician and palliative care physician. She has developed and evaluated a number of comprehensive clinical programs for seriously ill older adults, including inpatient and outpatient palliative care programs, community-based complex illness programs, and home-care medicine programs. She is director of Tideswell at University of California, San Francisco, in addition to serving as the Harris Fishbon Distinguished Professor in Clinical Translational Research and Aging at UCSF.

What we all need, she told me, are people who are local enough and who understand health systems and what they offer, to help us. One of Tideswell's initiatives has been to evaluate peer-delivery models, which is to train people in the community such as judges, police officers, and bankers, to identify elders who need services.

Obstacles to Progress

Many advocates call for funding the kind of social supports that will enable more elders to remain as autonomous as possible, for as long as possible, by achieving savings through high quality, coordinated care and avoiding unnecessary hospital readmissions, emergency visits, and excessive tests, treatments, and procedures. However, we must understand the magnitude of the likely resistance to major reconfigurations of Medicare and Medicaid policies.

If there's any doubt, think back to the storm of controversy over the made up "death panels" invoked in 2009. It has taken more than five years for lawmakers to survive the post-traumatic stress—and fear—this episode engendered. How did that happen? In its early stages, the Affordable Care Act was to include a provision that would have reimbursed physicians for periodically spending the time to talk with their patients about what kind of care patients envisioned at the end of life.

Opposition got rolling in mid-July 2009, when Betsy McCaughey, the former lieutenant governor of New York and a health care commentator, suggested that the plan would require elders to be told how to end their lives. On a radio show hosted by Fred Thompson, she said, "Congress would make it mandatory—absolutely require—that every five years people in Medicare have a required counseling session that will tell them how to end their life sooner."

Sarah Palin, who clearly had not lost her taste for making mischief after she and John McCain lost the national election in 2008, took to Facebook in August 2009 to rail against what she called the proposed "death panels." [5]

Conservatives quickly joined the bandwagon. Logic and facts did not win the day but fear, irrationality, and toxic politics did. The provision was scrapped from the legislation. It has taken until very recently for CMS to consider and ultimately enable—as of January 2016—reimbursing physicians for engaging in these conversations with their patients.

In March 2015 at the National Action Conference of the Institute of Medicine's Committee on Approaching Death, Patrick Conway, chief medical officer at the Centers for Medicare and Medicaid Services, said his agency would consider the American Medical Association's proposed codes for reimbursing advance-care planning discussions. Dr. Conway really set conference attendees' hearts aflutter, though, when he said he was excited about the Medicare Care Choices model (discussed in Chapter 12). If successful, he said CMS has the regulatory authority to expand it nationally.

"If you don't understand this as a political problem, you'll never solve it," Bruce Vladeck, PhD, told the large gathering of health care professionals at that IOM conference. [6]

Vladeck is senior advisor at Nexera, a subsidiary of the New York Hospital Association. He is also board chairman of the nonprofit Medicare Rights Center. From 1993–97, he

A Better Future and A Call to Action

was the administrator of the Health Care Financing Administration (now called the Centers for Medicare and Medicaid Services—or CMS).

Vladeck pointed out that Medicare has spent $200 billion less than the Congressional Budget Office's 10-year projections in 2004 yet none of that savings has gone back into the Medicare program—or for any other domestic purpose.

That there could be a fixed pile of money that can be reallocated for other purposes is a "nice idea but it's not going to work because others are going to get to those savings before you do," he said. "Over the last 20 years we have eviscerated domestic discretionary spending."

That both the terminally ill and the non-terminally ill lack sufficient support is a disgrace, he asserted. "We shouldn't try to cover that up by sneaking them into Medicare and Medicaid payments."

"We need to significantly change the hospice benefit and use that as leverage to clean up and reshape the hospice industry."

And then, he added, we must significantly strengthen new standards for participation by hospice agencies, and "enforce the hell out of them."

Vladeck would also do away with the hospice benefit in nursing homes. Instead, nursing homes should become capable of delivering high-quality, end-of-life care by themselves, and be adequately reimbursed for it.

When I spoke to Vladeck not long after the conference, he said, "CMS operates in geological time. It's a very complex system with highly educated people with an investment in the status quo. The problem is that people [advocating for change] give up halfway."

More can be done beyond governmental action, he said.

Critical to improving the future of care is educating, or re-educating doctors in how to communicate with patients such that patients receive accurate information, understand the likely course of their illnesses, and know what their options are.

"Dealing with emotionally intense situations is not an easy thing," he said. "Training is absolutely necessary." In order to provide accurate information, physicians must be knowledgeable about out-of-hospital services and supports, which many currently are not.

As was the case with public attitudes toward tobacco use, a change in public perception about care through the end of life will be pivotal.

A Call to Action

How do we get to a better future? It's up to us to play a key role. It seems to me that Tom Daschle's prescription for success—good public policy, superior technology, and enlightened leadership—is missing one element, and that is public engagement. Ira Byock put it this way: "Absent the emergence of a real consumer movement, we're toast."

Baby boomers may not be the Greatest Generation, but we have certainly proven ourselves to be the noisiest and most insistent—if not spectacularly self-absorbed—not

A Better Future and A Call to Action

only by sheer force of numbers but also by our penchant for questioning the received wisdom of older generations. We questioned war, racial inequality, sexual politics, and gender discrimination. We thought we invented sex. We rethought ground rules and role responsibilities in marriage. We railed against the medicalization of childbirth.

The more narcissistic of our generational traits will forge a path to invented rites and rituals around the end of life. Just as there are life coaches who help people figure out their personal and career issues and goals, and doulas who help women give birth, I expect that there will be a great many more end-of-life coaches to help ease people's transitions and doulas who will sit vigil for the dying. People will develop creative ways to review their lives, tell their stories, and share them with the world.

On a broader scale, as more of us age, Dr. Joanne Lynn said, "We will either wake up, have a painful set of debates, and come to better solutions, or we'll learn to not notice."

It is time not only for us to notice, but to get involved, time to use the collective strength of our loud and insistent voices to focus on aging issues. There are plenty of ways to do it.

The Center for Elder Care and Advanced Illness offers excellent resources on how to get involved in your community, at www.medicaring.org/action-guides/get-started. You'll find invaluable information about improving care transitions and, my personal favorite, the Agitator's Guide to Elder Care. http://medicaring.org/action-guides/agitators-guide/

Last Comforts

Among other activities, the guide urges us to attend debates or political candidate forums and raise our voices about elder care and caregiver support, share an experience and describe how the system might have made it better, easier, or more effective.

We can also campaign for an elder care improvement initiative on the policy agenda of the professional, consumer, disease-based, and volunteer groups with which we are involved.

We can tell our own stories—write responses to blogs, post stories on websites (such as www.medicaring.org), or talk with civic leaders. These stories should be tied to specific aspects of policy and practice.

A webinar on how to get involved with the Medicaring initiative in your community is available at https://altarum.adobeconnect.com/_a758956138/p1gikillyf8/.

To concentrate on the issue of culture change, a good place to start is the Pioneer Network, which offers a very useful community outreach toolkit at www.pioneernetwork.net/Consumers/InformTransformInspire.

LeadingAge, an association of 6,000 nonprofits dedicated to "making America a better place to grow old," offers guidance on advocacy and updates on proposed legislation aimed mainly at its membership. However, it is also a useful source for consumers and caregivers who want to be apprised about these issues. Its grassroots guidance is at http://www.leadingage.org/LeadingAge_Grassroots_Connector/.

The National Consumer Voice for Quality Long-Term Care offers policy resources and information, an advocacy toolkit, resident-directed care fact sheets, and a listing of citizen advocacy groups around the country. There may be one in your area. Check www.theconsumervoice.org.

To advocate for patient-centered care on the national level, look into the Patient Quality of Life Coalition. Formed in 2013, this group is one of the few that includes patients, caregivers, and survivors, as well as hospitals, health systems, hospices, physicians, nurses, social workers, chaplains, and researchers. See www.patientqualityoflife.org.

Joanne Lynn posed this question when I interviewed her: When issues of advanced illness, frailty, and care through the end of life become pressing, will elder boomers focus solely on their own interests or advocate for the group as a whole?

It's our choice, my friends, and the time for us to tap into those activism genes of ours once again, is now.

Coda

One of the exercises we did in hospice volunteer training was to write our own obituaries. We had to state our age and what we died of. An odd assignment, you might think, but thought-provoking nonetheless. After we wrote our obits, our group talked about how it made us feel. For me, it was weird but not particularly disconcerting. (For the record, I imagined being 90, done in from something from the cardiovascular menu, with my family by my side.)

The truth is I'm as hungry for life as ever and am no closer to wrapping my head around the fact of my mortality than I was after the deaths of my parents or even after years

Last Comforts

of being a hospice volunteer. Gradually, however, I recognize that I've begun thinking slightly differently than I did when I was younger. For one afternoon every year in May, for example, my husband and I do a pre-season pilgrimage to a beach club in Atlantic Beach on Long Island where my family had been members when I was growing up. It is my favorite beach. Every year, as we drive over the Atlantic Beach Bridge, catching a glimpse of the Atlantic Ocean, I am instantly happy. When we park in the parking lot nearest to where my family's cabana had been, I am happier still.

We walk the beach. We walk along the ocean for about a mile to a jetty overlooking the Rockaways. On the way back, we take the circuitous route past the club's huge pool and back to the row of cabanas where my family used to be. I am a homing pigeon; I could find it blindfolded. We enjoy a picnic lunch and lay out in our beach chairs for a while. Seagulls squawk. Kids play catch, as they have since I was a kid, while planes drone above us as they climb above the ocean, leaving from nearby John F. Kennedy Airport. (It was here that I saw the 747 jumbo jets for the first time, when they began flying. "Whales," my father called them, for their odd shape. Memories come easily here.)

On our walk, we'll usually see people getting ready for the summer season: sweeping out the sand that's accumulated over the winter, painting interiors, hanging wall decorations, maybe installing a new refrigerator. I've always felt a faint twinge of regret, knowing that we wouldn't be a part of the coming summer here. It wasn't until several years ago, though, that I began to wonder: whether that regret is a hint

A Better Future and A Call to Action

of what it feels like, to know in your gut that your life is coming to its end, and that life is going to continue, regardless of whether or not you are here. These sweet, momentary pleasures of feeling the cold waves on my feet along the shore, or my toes wiggling in the sand and my face warmed by the sun, are they never to be felt again?

It's difficult to contemplate. I think about my mother and how, even before the brain tumor changed her so radically, she began to withdraw. With a chorus of mundane chatter around her, she seemed focused elsewhere. Was she thinking, this will all be going on and I won't be here for it? I'd catch a glimpse of her and want to lasso her back, to keep her in our midst. Come back, Mom, don't leave us yet.

Perhaps it's human nature not to dwell on the idea of "this will go on and I won't be here."

My thoughts sometimes turn to whimsy. Maybe by the time I'm 90 I'll be able to recreate my beach pilgrimage through virtual reality: a headset that lets me "walk" the beach, wiggle toes in the sand, feel the sun on my face. Or maybe it will be possible to turn old photos into virtual reality and I'll be able to revisit the places my husband and I have loved the most. Maybe I'll be able to "swim" my mile in a virtual swimming pool, although I'd no doubt miss the pleasure of feeling real water around me.

How about this? Maybe I'll be able to "visit" with my parents again, or re-experience my son, my stepchildren, and my grandchildren growing up.

I could while away countless hours in virtual pursuits, without ever leaving couch or bed, until it would be time for my televised nurse case manager to check my status and make sure I'm comfortable. Maybe I'll have a robot companion to remind me to take medications. Maybe the robot will busy itself straightening my room, preparing a snack or, if I choose, purr like my cat if I feel the need to hold it for comfort.

Maybe after I'm gone, my friends and family will be able to visit me, say, if I were turned into a hologram. The technology exists, and it's not just available for special events like Michael Jackson "performing" at a music awards ceremony. [7]

Think of all the stories and advice I could share, available any time, although I imagine that after a while I'd be stored away and hauled out maybe once a year. Think of how weird but maybe comforting it might be, to create a hologram specifically to show at a memorial service—interacting with my family and friends. People do that in videos now, but I'm sure the 3D effect of a hologram would be awesome.

In our obituary-writing exercise, a few people in my group expected to die suddenly; or to go quietly in their sleep. Personally, I'd rather have a little advance notice that the end is coming. Here's why. I've been to more funerals and memorial services than I'd care to have gone to. I know you probably have too, and like me, you're always moved by what people say about the deceased. The anecdotes are funny and touching; the love and affection of family and friends are palpable. It's clear how cherished and appreciated the deceased had been, how unique and unforgettable, to so many of us. This is a comfort to the community of the mourning, perhaps.

A Better Future and A Call to Action

But the deceased does not hear it.

So, kids, here's what I want. If I'm lucky enough to have my advance notice and I still have my wits about me, I want to hear it before I go. I want to have a big party where people tell me I've been important to them; what they'll remember about me; maybe, what I've taught them; how they knew how much I loved them. And, for this one occasion, for those who are shy about speaking in public, I'm hoping you can take a deep breath and forge on. I promise, I will tell you, and will keep telling you, if I haven't driven you crazy by telling you all along regardless of illness, how precious you are to me, and what you have meant to me too. Which is: everything.

Chapter 13 Endnotes

1. healthaffairs.org/blog/2015/06/17/fifty-years-in-medi-care-has-transformed-health-care-whats-in-store-for-the-next-fifty/ Former Senate Majority Leader Tom Daschle is currently a lobbyist.

2. For more on CMS's seven quality measures for hospice: ww.cms.gov/Medicare/Quality-Initiatives-Patient-Assessment-Instruments/Hospice-Quality-Reporting/Current-Measures.html

3. "More Than a Meal" study www.mealsonwheelsamerica.org/theissue/facts-resources/more-than-a-meal

4. "Older Americans Act: Updated Information on Unmet Need for Services" GAO–15–601R: Jun 10, 2015. www.gao.gov/products/GAO-15-601R

5. Politifact called "death panels" the lie of the year in 2009: www.politifact.com/truth-o-meter/article/2009/dec/18/politifact-lie-year-death-panels/

6. Videos of all sessions of the IOM National Action conference on Policies and Payment Systems to Improve End of Life Care:
www.iom.edu/Activities/Aging/TransformingEndOfLife/2015-MAR-20/Videos/Welcome%20and%20Introductions/1-Welcome-Video.aspx

7. The technology already exists to make a hologram of yourself. www.aimholographics.com

Part Three

A Consumer's Guide to Navigating the Present

❝All I know is that first you've got to get mad. You've got to say, 'I'm a HUMAN BEING, God damn it! My life has VALUE!' So I want you to get up now. I want all of you to get up out of your chairs. I want you to get up right now and go to the window. Open it, and stick your head out, and yell, 'I'M AS MAD AS HELL, AND I'M NOT GO- ING TO TAKE THIS ANYMORE!' ❞ —Newscaster char- acter Howard Beale, Network, 1976.

Last Comforts

The state of end-of-life care in the U.S. is currently fragmented, dysfunctional, and costly. A yawning chasm exists between the care people say they want and the care they receive toward the end of life. Our future may be far better, but if you are dealing with a life-limiting illness, or caring for someone who is, the goal of this chapter is to help you navigate the choppy waters of our health-care system. It offers practical points about life-prolonging measures, documenting your goals in an advance directive, or a form of POLST, which is the acronym for Physician Orders for Life Sustaining Treatment.

Finally, this chapter addresses how to evaluate nursing homes, palliative care, and hospice.

Thinking About "The Big Three:" Feeding Tubes, CPR, Mechanical Ventilation

How can you protect yourself from futile treatments, cascading complications, and an unpeaceful end? Take steps before you reach a crisis. Think deeply about what you want. Then talk it over with the people you trust most to represent you. Document your goals and preferences in an advance directive.

I cannot say it better than James Salwitz, medical oncologist, who has written in his Sunrise Rounds blog: "Cancers spread, coronary arteries close, sudden pneumonias invade. Doctors see the medical future through a haze, and even the most empathetic cannot read your soul... Therefore, the final burden for each decision, for setting goals, for balancing personal benefit and cost, comes back to the patient. It requires forethought, discussion, and education. It demands introspection; what are your dreams, priorities, and limits? Who are you? What do you want? It requires planning, now, today, when you are still hopefully healthy, well before the moment of critical decision."

Can you know what you really want without understanding the mechanics of what I would call the "big three"—feeding tubes, CPR, and mechanical ventilation? I freely admit my bias against having these measures taken for me unless there is a good chance that the circumstances requiring them are deemed temporary and there's an equally good chance of recovering mentally, if not entirely physically. But I would not judge anyone harshly for wanting all possible measures taken to prolong life. I do believe being better informed about them is important, though. Here are some starting points for your own pursuit of information:

On CPR

In the mid-1970s, standards for CPR from the National Conference for Cardiopulmonary Resuscitation and Emergency Cardiac Care, published in the Journal of the American Medical Association, recognized that CPR should not be used in certain situations, such as "cases of terminal irreversible illness when death is not unexpected. Resuscitation in these circumstances may represent a positive violation of a person's right to die with dignity." But now, unless you have instructed otherwise, application of CPR is standard procedure for cardiac or respiratory failure.

As mentioned in Chapter 9, physicians' own preferences at the end-of-life, overwhelmingly include a resounding "no thanks" to CPR and other so-called "heroic" measures. They know too well the potential harmful effects: broken ribs, lung or spleen punctured from the force applied, the possibility of brain damage if patients have been without oxygen for too long—with care escalating to being placed on a mechanical ventilator.

In an article in The Health Care Blog, Ken Murray, MD wrote: "When applied to a patient in the last stages of a terminal decline, CPR is particularly ineffective." [1]

He referenced a 2010 study in the journal Supportive Care in Cancer. It looked at terminal patients who wanted no CPR but got it anyway. Of the 69 patients studied, eight regained a pulse, but 48 hours later, all were dead.

"Well-meaning CPR advocates talk in terms of 'survival,' he said, but all the term means is that the heart again beats on its own. In the study of 69 patients discussed in the journal Supportive Care in Cancer, survival was 11 percent, but survival—in the sense of regaining a reasonable quality of life—was zero."

On Feeding Tubes

There are two types of feeding tubes. A nasogastric tube is inserted through the nose and into the stomach through the esophagus. The gastronomy tube, sometimes called a percutaneous endoscopic gastrostomy (PEG) tube, is inserted surgically into the stomach through the skin. Liquid nutrition, water, and medications can be poured into the tube or pumped by a mechanical device. They are for patients who lose the ability to swallow or cannot eat and drink enough by mouth.

Some of the potential problems that can arise with feeding tubes are pneumonia (if the tube is displaced, or if regurgitated food enters the lungs); infections or ulcers; patients damaging themselves by removing the tubes.

The Society for Post-Acute and Long-Term Care Medicine addressed this issue in its "10 Things Physicians and Patients Should Question" on the Choosing Wisely website at http://www.choosingwisely.org/societies/amda-the-society-for-post-acute-and-long-term-care-medicine/. Essentially, they say, for people with advanced dementia, "Don't" offer assistance with feeding. I consider that advice equally pertinent for people who are in the end stage of a terminal illness.

To have conversations with their providers, patients need better information about what care they truly need. Recognizing this, Consumer Reports and the American Board of Internal Medicine (ABIM) Foundation developed the Choosing Wisely website. Its goal is to help consumers choose care that is supported by evidence; that does not duplicate tests or procedures previously received; and that is truly necessary. Additional information is available at www.

consumerhealthchoices.org. It includes advice for caregivers, and treatments and tests for seniors.

According to the Society for Post-Acute and Long-Term Care Medicine:

Strong evidence exists that artificial nutrition does not prolong life or improve quality of life in patients with advanced dementia. Substantial functional decline and recurrent or progressive medical illnesses may indicate that a patient who is not eating is unlikely to obtain any significant or long-term benefit from artificial nutrition.

Feeding tubes are often placed after hospitalization, frequently with concerns for aspirations, and for those who are not eating. Contrary to what many people think, tube feeding does not ensure the patient's comfort or reduce suffering; it may cause fluid overload, diarrhea, abdominal pain, local complications, less human interaction and may increase the risk of aspiration.

Assistance with oral feeding is an evidence-based approach to provide nutrition for patients with advanced dementia and feeding problems.

On Mechanical Ventilation

There are good reasons to have mechanical ventilation, either during surgery, or for a short period to allow the patient's body to rest and recover from injury, infection or an illness like pneumonia. I think about Steve Saling, living with ALS thanks to outstanding care and to the ventilator that breathes for him. It's quite another matter toward the end of life, though.

A Consumer's Guide

Here's what's involved: a tube is inserted through the mouth, into the windpipe. It is connected to a ventilator, which pushes air into your lungs. You will be in the intensive care unit in the hospital. You won't be able to speak, or eat. You will need frequent tests. If you're uncomfortable and anxious, you may try to pull the tube out. That may result in your being sedated, or having your hands tied down. There is a risk of lung infection.

Let's say you have chronic obstructive pulmonary disease (COPD) and can no longer breathe on your own. The University of Ottawa prepared a workbook for patients with COPD to help them make decisions about their care. It is available at https://decisionaid.ohri.ca/docs/das/COPD.pdf. Of 100 people who choose intubation and mechanical ventilation, 20 will never come off the ventilator and will die in the hospital. Another 10 will come off the ventilator but will die in the hospital. Thirty will come off the ventilator and survive for at least one year, while 40 will come off the ventilator and die within a year.

One of my favorite books about end-of-life care is the short but eminently practical *Hard Choices for Loving People* by Hank Dunn, a hospice chaplain. He makes the point that the uncomfortable side effects of having a tube inserted down the windpipe, or surgically connected through the throat directly into the windpipe, are "acceptable to most people because the tube and ventilator are removed as soon as the need for them is gone." He acknowledges "the fear of not being able to breathe can be just as great as the shortness of breath itself."

"But some patients who have a long history of the disease that causes respiratory failure… may have to face the possibility that once they are placed on the ventilator they may not be able to get off again," he writes. "Your physician can help you assess whether or not the use of the ventilator is likely to be temporary or permanent."

Talking the Talk

Much of the discussion about end-of-life issues these days revolves around the importance of The Conversation—that difficult discussion we never want to have, but must have with our family, friends, or health care proxy. If we had a limited amount of time left to live, what would be most important to us? What would make life continue to be worth living? What would we be willing to tolerate, in terms of rigorous and aggressive treatment, in order to achieve a longer life? If we have just received a diagnosis of dementia, how would we want to advise those who will be caring for us when we could no longer articulate our preferences?

We can't just talk about this once. As our circumstances change, our feelings, values and wishes are likely to change too. Document your wishes. The people you hold near and dear may suffer the pain of impending loss—it's hard enough to bear under the best of circumstances—but you can give them the gift of sparing them the added burden of guessing what path to pursue. You can spare them feeling guilty about second-guessing their decisions for you. You can short-circuit a toxic brew of family dissension that would otherwise poison

A Consumer's Guide

family relationships for years to come, when family members cannot agree among themselves about how best to manage your care.

How do you even begin to broach this subject with your family, your family-of-choice, or your friends? One good source to guide you is The Conversation Project. This non-profit, begun in 2010, is led by the columnist Ellen Goodman. Responsible for her mother's care at the end of her life, Goodman had no idea what her mother might have wanted because they never discussed it. Complicating matters was that her mother had dementia. When there were "cascading decisions to make," as Goodman explains in a video on the organization's website, she felt unprepared and blindsided.

Goodman's experience is not unique.

To kick off the discussion, the organization offers a handy "starter kit," available at www.theconversationproject. org/starter-kit/intro/.

There's even a game to play to get the discussion started. Called "My Gift of Grace" it sells for $24.95. It comes in a box with an instruction sheet, 47 question cards, and 24 thank you chips. Anyone can play; and its makers say the game can take 20 minutes to three hours, depending on the discussion. During each turn, all the players have a chance to share their answers to the same question—such as, "If you had to pick one person to share an anecdote about you at your memorial service, who would that be?"

Another is this. "What three non-medical facts about you should your doctors know, in order for them to give you the best possible care?" The game is at www.mygiftofgrace. com.

Since it is not uncommon for siblings or others entrusted with the care of an aging or ill parent or relative to clash over that care, some have turned to professional mediators for assistance. The Association for Conflict Resolution has an ACR elder decision-making section, which at this writing has 230 members nationwide. To find a mediator in your area, visit www.acreldersection.weebly.com.

Of course, you cannot plan for every eventuality. Illness has a way of forging surprising, unanticipated, and unexpected paths. Innumerable things can go awry. What about antibiotics if you develop infection? Fevers? What about catheterization? In cardiac care, is there ever a right time to remove pacemakers or left-ventricle assist devices? The answers may not be clear-cut.

Regardless of whether you are terminally ill or whether the medical devices prolong life, you have the right to request their withdrawal. If you cannot speak for yourself, your health care proxy can. You may run into resistance from a physician about it. In that case, the physician should help you find a colleague who will not object to carrying out your wishes.

When the path ahead is not clear, here is where it helps to be able to talk openly and honestly with your medical team. Your team should accord you the time and patience the discussion requires, outlining next steps for you to consider. If your team has not already recommended it, ask for a palliative care consultation to help you sort through the complexities of the benefits and risks of care in light of how you want to live the rest of your life.

Advance Directives

When you are not able to speak for yourself, an advance directive and a designated health care proxy will help your family and friends navigate the system more smoothly, on your behalf. You don't need a lawyer to have one. Bear in mind it is still possible for these documents to fall between the cracks (as was true in my father's case described in Chapter 1). It is possible that even if your primary care physician has a copy of your advance directive, the specialists who tend to you as disease progresses or a medical crisis ensues, do not. Either you or your proxy should not be reticent in reminding physicians, administrators, or whoever is in charge of your care, that these documents exist.

Fortunately, there are several sources for advance directive templates. One of the more popular is Five Wishes, created by the nonprofit, Aging With Dignity at http://www. agingwithdignity.org/forms/5wishes.pdf

Five Wishes developed the document in 1997 and distributed it with support from a grant by the Robert Wood Johnson Foundation. Five Wishes Online was introduced in 2011, allowing people to complete Five Wishes on screen and to print out a personalized document immediately. It is a popular tool written in plain English that can be used as a legal document in most states. It is also available in more than 28 languages.

Last Comforts

Another useful source is Caring Connections, a program of the National Hospice and Palliative Care Organization (NHPCO). You can find advance directive forms for each state at http://www.caringinfo.org/i4a/pages/index.cfm?pageid=3289.

Unlike Five Wishes, which charges a small fee, Caring Connections makes its forms available free of charge. Depending on your state's requirements, you may or may not need to have two witnesses sign the document, or to have it notarized.

There is an app for advance care planning, too. My Health Care Wishes, from the American Bar Association's Commission on Law and Aging, includes a health-care wishes overview and a section for your advance-care plan documents, either in pdf or Word format. The documents can be stored on your smartphone or tablet. (The data is not stored on a server or cloud.)

The app enables you to include family and medical contacts, insurance, and other health-related information. In case of an emergency, the information can be emailed to the appropriate health care providers. You can also store information for, say, an elder parent, who will get the app's wallet ID card with your contact information. In an emergency, medical staff can reach you and you can text, fax or email your parent's advance care directive.

This begs the question, of course: why not just store documents for yourself or your elder parent on a file storage service like DropBox, or give your parent your own "in case of emergency" wallet card?

A Consumer's Guide

It's POLST Time

Let's say you are among the minority in this country who has a written advance care planning document. You've designated someone close to you to be your health-care proxy. What more do you need? If you've just been diagnosed with a serious illness (and a health-care professional would not be surprised if you died within a year) it's time to think about POLST. That stands for Physician Orders for Life Sustaining Treatment. (Depending on the state, these orders are also known by other acronyms, including POST, MOST and MOLST, to name a few.)

The main difference between an advance care document and POLST is that the POLST is an actionable medical order. It becomes part of your medical record and is valid in all care settings, whether you are at home, in a hospital, or in a rehab or nursing facility.

It is also different from an advance directive because it's applicable to people of any age. That compares with advance directives, available only to those over 18.

The Physician Orders for Life Sustaining Treatment outlines medical orders for current treatment (as compared to future possibilities). It guides actions by emergency medical personnel (who will do everything they can to keep you alive unless your POLST document specifies otherwise). And it guides inpatient treatment. The form must be completed and signed by a health-care professional (such as a physician or advanced practice nurse). Although the document cannot be filled out by a patient, the answers are, of course, based on discussion with the consumer. It does have to be signed by a professional.

Susan Tolle, MD, director of the Center for Ethics in Health Care at the Oregon Health and Science University, is credited with leading the effort to put the physician's orders for life-sustaining treatment in writing. She is also responsible for developing the National POLST Paradigm Task Force (NPPTF) with colleagues in the late 1990s. States implement their own versions of this form; the task force's role is to promote the idea, although it does endorse documents created by the states. Oregon and West Virginia were the first to create forms for these medical orders. NPPTF has endorsed documents in 13 other states. All states except Alabama, Alaska, Iowa, Mississippi, Nebraska, Oklahoma, and South Dakota have developed their own (though many have not been endorsed by the task force). To find out the status in your state, visit www.polst.org.

The Physician Orders for Life Sustaining Treatment is based on discussion with the consumer, and is therefore all about consumer goals and preferences.

The New Jersey Practitioner Orders for Life-Sustaining Treatment (POLST) is a deceptively simple document, a one-pager that asks about your goals of care; what you want in the way of medical interventions (full treatment, limited treatment, symptom treatment only); artificially administered fluids and nutrition; CPR; airway management (if you are in respiratory distress and still have a pulse); and your surrogate. Here's the kicker: you don't have to fill out the entire form. (These are tough questions and it may take more than a couple of minutes to make, literally life-and-death decisions). But, if you leave any section blank, it implies that you want full treatment for issues related to that section.

The 'goals of care' section advises the physician or nurse practitioner to ask the simple question: "What are your hopes for the future?" It lists such examples as longevity; cure; remission; better quality of life; desire to attend an upcoming family event; to live without pain, nausea, or shortness of breath; eating, driving, gardening, enjoying time with grandchildren. The section provides about an inch of space to delineate these goals. Most people I know, myself included, could probably fill at least a page, single-spaced, if not more.

What Palliative Care Should Look Like

Surprisingly, many people do not know what palliative care is despite its great strides in recent years. A Consumer Reports survey of more than 2,000 adults, for example, showed that 61 percent had never heard of palliative care. In an intensive care unit, the goal of palliative care is to alleviate stress, to identify goals of care, to make medical decisions aligned with the goals of care and to provide important to information patients and families, Jessica Nutik Zitter, MD explained. But Nutik Zitter, who is board certified in both critical care and palliative care, added, "This just doesn't happen a lot in the ICU."

As the population ages and the demand for palliative care grows, the ability to assess quality throughout the country and across care settings is increasingly important. Dr. Joseph Rotella is chief medical officer of the American Academy of Hospice and Palliative Medicine (AAHPM). He also co-chairs its 'measuring what matters clinical user panel.' Rotella explained that because there has been "no consistency regarding which measures are required by various groups, from accrediting organizations to payers," AAHPM and the Hospice and Palliative Nurses Association (HPNA) came up with quality indicators for "measuring what matters."

"There has not been enough focus on cultural sensitivity and social supports. The quality indicators represent a small set of measures to use right now in hospice and palliative care because they are meaningful to patients and have a real impact on them," he said.

Developing these measures was a rigorous process. It started with appointing co-chairs from each organization and additional co-chairs for the clinical user panel, staff people from AAHPM and HPNA, 11 members on the technical advisory panel, 27 members on the clinical user panel (including social workers and grief counselors) and a quality committee. The preliminary measures were sent to other organizations for comment. Hundreds of people had a chance to comment.

The 10 Measures

1. Seriously ill palliative care and hospice patients receive a comprehensive assessment (physical, psychological, social, spiritual, and functional) soon after admission.

A Consumer's Guide

2. Seriously ill palliative care and hospice patients are screened for pain, shortness of breath, nausea, and constipation during the admission visit.

3. Seriously ill palliative care and hospice patients who screen positive for at least moderate pain receive medication or other treatment within 24 hours.

4. Patients with advanced or life-threatening illness are screened for shortness of breath and, if positive, to at least a moderate degree, have a plan to manage it.

5. Seriously ill palliative care and hospice patients have a documented discussion regarding emotional needs.

6. Hospice patients have a documented discussion of spiritual concerns or preference not to discuss them.

7. Seriously ill palliative care and hospice patients have documentation of the surrogate decision-maker's name (such as the person who has health-care power of attorney) and contact information, or absence of a surrogate.

8. Seriously ill palliative care and hospice patients have documentation of their preferences for life-sustaining treatments.

9. Vulnerable elders with documented preferences to withhold or withdraw life-sustaining treatments have their preferences followed.

10. Palliative care and hospice patients, or their families, are asked about their experience of care using a relevant survey.

Dr. Rotella told me that AAHPM and HPNA are hoping that palliative and hospice programs will voluntarily adopt these measures. They were not designed to be an accountability program and the organizations are not recommending to the Centers for Medicare and Medicaid Services that they become mandatory.

About Nursing Homes

How do you find out about the quality of care in a nursing home? Medicare's Nursing Home Compare website http://www.medicare.gov/nursinghomecompare is a good place to start, although you should consider it just a starting point. You can also find comparisons for home health agencies on the Medicare website, at https://www.medicare.gov/homehealthcompare/.

The government rates nursing homes on a scale of one to five, with five being the best grade (though it stresses that these ratings are not meant to be guidelines, standards of care, or an endorsement). Ratings are based on health inspections, overall staffing, and quality of care. In all it looks at about 180 separate aspects of care, including information on falls, pressure ulcers, weight loss, loss of continence, and use of antipsychotic drugs.

Its health inspection process is based on visits by trained surveyors (inspectors). Federal inspectors check on the work of state inspectors to make sure they're following national regulations, and that any differences among states stay within reasonable bounds. Staffing and quality information, by contrast, is based on data provided by the nursing homes themselves.

Staffing data are reported just once a year and reflect

staffing over a two-week period. It is entirely possible that staffing could be boosted prior to reporting requirements and reduced later. Medicare advises that quality is generally better in nursing homes that have more staff who work directly with residents and that it's important to ask nursing homes about their staffing levels, the qualifications of their staff, and the staff turnover rate. Ask also how long it takes to replace staff who leave.

The quality ratings look at the overall number of staff (registered nurses, licensed practical nurses, licensed vocational nurses, certified nursing assistants) compared to the number of residents. They also measure the number of hours staff members spend with each patient. The ratings consider differences in how sick the nursing home residents are in each nursing home, since that will make a difference in how many staff members are needed. Quality measures show how well the nursing home helps people keep their ability to dress and eat, or how well the nursing home prevents and treats pressure ulcers. Medicare advises having a discussion with the nursing home staff about these measures of quality care. Ask what else they're doing to improve the care they give their residents.

Deeply buried in the Nursing Home Compare website is an excellent 56-page booklet from Medicare, called "Your Guide to Choosing a Nursing Home or Other Long-Term Care." It is available at http://www.medicare.gov/Pubs/pdf/02174.pdf. The guide stresses the importance of visiting prospective nursing homes—more than once—and offers very specific questions to ask while you're there about every aspect of staffing, operations, and care.

Last Comforts

The guide provides a handy checklist to bring when you nursing homes. It also outlines your rights as a nursing home resident. It advises that you may ask to attend a meeting of a resident council or family council to understand how the nursing home responds to resident and family concerns. The guide also suggests contacting your state health department or state licensing agency for full copies of nursing home surveys, or copies of the most recent complaint investigation reports.

To Medicare's comprehensive guide, I would add a few additional questions, particularly regarding care for people with dementia. What is a nursing home's approach to comfort care? Does it initiate family meetings to establish goals of care for residents and work with residents and families on advance directives? Does it explain the availability of palliative care? Does it offer or require additional training for certified nursing assistants who provide most of the direct care for nursing home residents? I'd certainly ask about their views about culture change.

What is Culture Change?

The Pioneer Network defines culture change as "the national movement for the transformation of older adult services, based on person-directed values and practices where the voices of elders and those working with them are considered and respected. Core person-directed values are choice, dignity, respect, self-determination, and purposeful living."

Assisted living developments are not regulated as comprehensively as are skilled nursing facilities. Yet the people moving into assisted living developments are older and sicker than was the case years ago. The Pioneer Network offers a list of excellent questions to ask if you're considering a move to assisted living. You want to make sure it offers patient-centered care. The list is at www.pioneernetwork.net/data/documents/keyquestions-assistedliving.pdf.

About Dementia

The Greater Illinois Chapter of the Alzheimer's Association offers a useful—and free—online resource, "Encouraging Comfort Care: A Guide for Families of People with Dementia Living in Care Facilities." Funded by the Retirement Research Foundation, this 21-page booklet provides information for families and staffers at long-term care facilities. The booklet discusses Alzheimer's disease and related dementias, particularly care issues related to the late and final stages.

The guide helps clarify the kinds of medical decisions they may face on behalf of loved ones with dementia living in nursing homes, assisted living facilities, and other types of care facilities. It offers a checklist of comfort care measures to be discussed with staff members of care facilities. The guide is at http://www.alzheimers-illinois.org/pti/comfort_care_guide.asp.

On its website, the dementia program at Hospice of the Valley in Scottsdale, Arizona, offers outstanding information for caregivers about communicating with loved ones with dementia. It addresses understanding behaviors and the different stages of the disease, as well as excellent practical advice about medications (particularly, what types of medications should not be given to people with dementia). It tackles issues in making health-care decisions. Its short and effective educational videos are at https://www.hov.org/educational-videos.

The National Institute on Aging of the National Institutes of Health offers tip sheets, resources, and links for caregivers in its Alzheimer's Disease Education and Referral Center. The website includes valuable information about middle- and late-stage illness, legal matters, and how caretakers can take care of their own health. These resources are at https://www.nia.nih.gov/alzheimers/topics/caregiving.

Debunking Some Myths About Hospice

Although hospice has been around for more than 40 years, it is still enshrouded in mystery for many. Here are some common misconceptions.

1. Myth: Hospice is a place. Hospice services and benefits are available wherever people are most comfortable and for most, that means their own homes. A small percentage of people are cared for in freestanding hospice facilities. Hospice care is also available to people in nursing homes.

2. Myth: If you choose hospice care, it means you're giving up on life and hope. Hospice care aims to enable you to live the fullest and most comfortable life possible, as long as possible. For many, it means the luxury of time you can spend focusing on your life, your family and friends, with-

out the physical and emotional challenges and distractions of continued treatments, clinic visits and hospitalizations. With good pain management and control of symptoms (such as fatigue, coughs, constipation or lack of appetite) people can experience greater comfort and a sense of well-being.

3. Myth: Hospice is only for cancer patients. Although it had its roots in caring for advanced cancer patients, hospice care is appropriate for people with any type of life-limiting illness, such as heart failure, COPD, kidney failure or advanced dementia. Under current regulations, if your illness is expected to be fatal within six months if it runs its natural course, you would be eligible for hospice care.

4. Myth: Once you make the decision to enter hospice care, you cannot change your mind. You can opt out of hospice care any time. So if you decide to try curative treatment, for example, you may leave hospice care. And you can decide to be readmitted later on, after you've opted out.

5. Myth: You will be discharged from hospice care if you live longer than six months. As long as hospice can certify that your illness is still fatal and that you continue to decline, you can be re-certified for additional hospice care. But you can be discharged if you hit a "plateau" and are no longer declining (a live discharge).

6. Myth: Only Medicare-eligible people enroll in hospice. Hospice services are available for people of all ages, including, sadly, children with fatal diseases. Medicare pays for hospice benefits, including visits by nurses, health aides, social workers and chaplains, plus drugs related to the illness and equipment, such as commodes and hospital beds, that people

may need. Many health insurance policies for those under age 65 offer similar benefits. Medicare also pays for hospice services in assisted living and nursing home settings, although it does not pay for your rent or room and board.

Choosing a Hospice

Not all hospices are created equal. Although there is not yet a hospice equivalent to the Nursing Home Compare information, one is in the works. Meanwhile, the National Hospice and Palliative Care Organization presents helpful advice through its Caring Connections program. It suggests questions to ask when considering a hospice. A worksheet is available at http://www.caringinfo.org/files/public/brochures/Choosing_Hospice.pdf.

Contact your state health department or state licensing agency for full copies of hospice surveys, or copies of the most recent complaint investigation reports.

Chapter 14 Endnote

1. Ken Murray, MD. "How Doctors Die" Aug 6, 2012 the-healthcareblog.com/blog/2012/08/06/how-doctors-die/

Appendix A

Resources and Links

Bibliography

Brody, Jane. *Jane Brody's Guide to the Great Beyond: A Practical Primer to Help You and Your Loved Ones Prepare Medically, Legally, and Emotionally for the End of Life*. New York: Random House, 2009.

Brown, Theresa. *Critical Care: A New Nurse Faces Death, Life, and Everything in Between*. New York: HarperCollins, 2011.

Brown, Theresa. *The Shift: One Nurse, Twelve Hours, Four Patients' Lives*. New York: Algonquin Books, 2015.

Butler, Katy. *Knocking on Heaven's Door: The Path to a Better Way of Death*. New York: Simon & Schuster, 2013.

Byock Ira. *The Best Care Possible: A Physician's Quest to Transform Care through the End of Life*. New York: Penguin Publishing, 2013.

Byock, Ira. *Dying Well: Peace and Possibilities at the End of Life*. New York: Riverhead Books, 1998.

Last Comforts

Chast, Roz. *Can't We Talk About Something More Pleasant?* New York: Bloomsbury USA, 2014.

Dunn, Hank. *Hard Choices for Loving People.* Lansdowne, PA: A & A Publishers Inc., Fifth edition, 2009.

Gawande, Atul. *Being Mortal: Medicine and What Matters in the End.* New York: Metropolitan Books, 2014.

Institute of Medicine. Committee on Approaching Death. *Dying in America: Improving Quality and Honoring Individual Preferences Near the End of Life.* Washington, DC: The National Academies Press, 2015.

Kiernan, Stephen P. *Last Rights: Rescuing the End of Life from the Medical System.* New York: St. Martin's Press, 2006.

Lynn, Joanne, Joan K. Harrold, and Janice Lynch Schuster. *Handbook for Mortals: Guidance for People Facing Serious Illnesses.* New York: Oxford University Press, 2011.

Manheimer, Eric. *Twelve Patients: Life and Death at Bellevue Hospital.* New York: Hachette Book Group, 2012.

Nuland, Sherwin B. *How We Die: Reflections on Life's Final Chapter.* New York: Vintage Books, 1995.

Oliver, David H. and Deborah Oliver. *Exit Strategy: Depriving Death of Its Strangeness.* Los Gatos: Smashwords, 2013.

Thomas, MD, Bill. *Second Wind: Navigating the Passage to a Slower, Deeper, and More Connected Life.* New York: Simon & Schuster, 2014.

Appendix A

Sweet, Victoria. *God's Hotel: A Doctor, a Hospital, and a Pilgrimage to the Heart of Medicine.* New York: Riverhead Books, 2012.

Volandes, MD, Angelo. *The Conversation: A Revolutionary Plan for End-of-Life Care.* New York: Bloomsbury USA, 2015.

Blogs and Newsletters

CoverAGE newsletter. www.Aging 2.com/newsletter: Aging 2.0, an organization where the mission is to accelerate innovation to improve the lives of older adults. Publishes this online newsletter about global technology and design innovations.

David's Cancer Videoblog. Dbocancerjourney.blogspot.com. The late David B. Oliver and his wife Debbie Oliver chronicle David's experiences, life lessons, and philosophy as his cancer progressed.

End of Life Decisions. www.Hankdunn.com. A hospice chaplain, Hank Dunn offers eminently practical advice and compassionate commentary on making difficult choices through the end of life.

GeriPal. A Geriatrics and Palliative Care Blog: www.Geripal. org. A forum for discussion, recent news, research, and free-thinking commentary.

Last Comforts

Get Palliative Care. www.getpalliativecare.org/blog/ The Center to Advance Palliative Care. Blog at Get Palliative Care provides excellent guidance, resources, and links for consumers with advanced serious illness. The blog tells the stories of how palliative care has helped people with serious illnesses.

Health AGEnda. http://www.jhartfound.org/blog/ The John Hartford Foundation apprises readers about its philanthropic work in aging health issues and innovations.

Hospice and Nursing Homes: www.hospiceand nursing-homes.blogspot.com. Frances Shani Parker, eldercare consultant, writes this blog. Topics include eldercare, hospice, nursing homes, caregiving, dementia, death, bereavement, and older adults in general.

Medical Futility. www.Medicalfutility.blogspot.com. Attorney and law professor Thaddeus Pope tracks judicial, legislative, policy and academic developments concerning medical futility and the limits on individual autonomy at the end of life.

KevinMD. www.kevinmd.com: An internal medicine physician, Kevin Pho founded and edits this blog, where more than 2,000 primary care doctors, surgeons, specialist physicians, nurses, medical students, policy experts, and patients share insights and commentary.

My Demented Mom. www.mydementedmom.com. Kathy Ritchie's often harrowing account of her mother's frontotemporal dementia. Ritchie calls it a site for young adult caregivers struggling and coping with "the long goodbye."

Appendix A

Next Avenue: www.nextavenue.org. News, information and advice to help people 50+ in navigating the rest of their lives, from the Public Broadcast Service (PBS).

OK to Die: www.OKtodie.com. Monica Williams-Murphy, MD, is an emergency room physician whose mission is to help people plan ahead, make their peace, and understand that it is OK to die naturally, and to make educated choices to die peacefully and comfortably.

Order of the Good Death. www.Orderofthegooddeath.com. Droll, bemused yet with great heart, Caitlin Doughty, a mortician, talks all things death-related in her blog and videos. She is great company.

Pallimed: A Hospice and Palliative Medicine Blog: www.pallimed.org. Tracks notable articles relevant to palliative care from a variety of journals but also includes reviewing media coverage of hospice and palliative care issues.

Pulse—Voices from the Heart of Medicine: www.pulse-voices.org. An online narrative medicine publication, Pulse publishes a personal story of illness and healing, told by and for health care professionals and non-professionals, every Friday. It also publishes art and poetry.

Sunrise Rounds:Health & Medicine Through the Eyes of a Medical Oncologist: www.sunriserounds.com. Often eloquent, always informative, and thought-provoking, James C. Salwitz writes movingly about advanced serious illness, caregiving, the health care system and end-of-life issues.

Videos and Webcasts

Webcast of the Institute of Medicine's Committee on Approaching Death's March 2015 National Action Conference:

http://www.iom.edu/Activities/Aging/
TransformingEndOfLife/2015-MAR-20/Videos/Welcome%20and%20Introductions/1-Welcome-Video.aspx

Atul Gawande, author of *Being Mortal,* gives the 19th annual Douglas West Endowed Memorial Lecture in Geriatrics and Palliative Care, Mt. Sinai Health System, April 15, 2015: https://www.youtube.com/watch?v=wrS_5vPQER0&feature=share

Atul Gawande, MD, Interview transcript, PBS/ Frontline: "Hope is Not a Plan: When Doctors, Patients, Talk Death," Feb. 10, 2015.
http://www.pbs.org/wgbh/pages/frontline/health-science-technology/being-mortal/dr-atul-gawande-hope-is-not-a-plan-when-doctors-patients-talk-death/

Jessica Nutik Zitter, MD, speaks about the need for palliative care in the ICU in a presentation, "All That Glitters," the Ungerleider Palliative Care Lecture Series at California Pacific Medical Center in San Francisco, April 6, 2015. https://www.youtube.com/watch?v=mdu8BbIr9uM&feature=youtu.be

Reporter Sean Cole reprises his Radiolab podcast, "The Bitter End" for NYU's Love and Let Die Symposium, in which doctors reveal how and why doctors don't want any heroic

efforts expended on their own behalf at the end of life.
Dr. Joseph Gallo and Dr. Ken Murray, June 18, 2013.
https://www.youtube.com/watch?v=m6e4_Guqsew

Steve Shields, CEO of Action Pact, talks about a new concept
in senior living in Liberty, Missouri: https://www.youtube.
com/watch?v=XivROF3a0MI

Overview of the Landscape of Advanced Illness and Long Term Care

http://www.thectac.org/wp-content/uploads/2014/10/
Advanced-Illness-Key-Statistics-12-22-2012.pdf

About long-term care: From the Centers for Disease Control
and Prevention:
http://www.cdc.gov/nchs/data/nsltcp/long_term_care_ser-
vices_2013.pdf

Hospice statistics: NHPCO Facts & Figures
Hospice Care in America: www.NHPCO.org

Palliative care statistics
www.capc.org, getpalliativecare.org

About Alzheimer's
and other types of dementia

http://www.nia.nih.gov/alzheimers/publication/alzheimers-disease-fact-sheet

http://www.nia.nih.gov/alzheimers

http://www.alzheimers.gov/

http://www.alz.org/we_can_help_24_7_helpline.asp

https://www.hov.org/dementia-program

https://www.hov.org/educational-videos

Organizations

Alzheimer's Association
www.alz.org

Alzheimer's Association, New York Chapter
www.alznyc.org

American Academy of Hospice and Palliative Medicine
www.aahpm.org

American Geriatrics Society
www.americangeriatrics.org

Center to Advance Palliative Care
www. capc.org

Center for Elder Care and Advanced Illness
www.altarum.org

Coalition to Transform Advanced Care
www.thectac.org

Appendix A

The Eden Alternative
www.edenalt.org

Elder Care Workforce Alliance
www.eldercareworkforce.org

Green House Project
www.greenhouseproject.org

Hospice and Palliative Nurses Association
www.HPNA.advancingexpertcare.org

Institute of Medicine
www.IOM.edu

LeadingAge
www.leadingage.org

National Hospice and Palliative Care Organization
www.NHPCO.org

PACE (Program of All-Inclusive Care for the Elderly)
www.pace4you.org

Patient Quality of Life Coalition
www.patientqualityoflife.org

PCORI (Patient-Centered Outcomes Research Institute)
www.pcori.org

Pioneer Network
www.pioneernetwork.net

SAGE (Services and Advocacy for GLBT Elders)
www.sageusa.org

Appendix B

Acronyms

AACN: American Association of Colleges of Nursing

AAHPM: American Academy of Hospice and Palliative Medicine

ABIM: American Board of Internal Medicine

ABMS: American Board of Medical Specialties

ACGME: Accreditation Council for Gradual Medical Education

ACR: Association for Conflict Resolution

ADCW: Advanced Direct Care Worker

ADLs: Activities of Daily Living (bathing, grooming, dressing, feeding, toileting, transferring, e.g., from bed to wheelchair)

ADN: Associate Degree in Nursing

AGS: American Geriatrics Society

ALS: Amyotrophic lateral sclerosis (Lou Gehrig's disease)

AMDA: The Society for Post-Acute and Long-Term Care

APRN: Advanced practice nurse practitioner

BSN: Bachelor of Science in Nursing

CAPC: Center to Advance Palliative Care

CBO: Congressional Budget Office

Last Comforts

CCTP: Community-Based Care Transitions Program

CDC: Centers for Disease Control and Prevention

CECAI: Center for Elder Care and Advanced Illness

CMMI: CMS's Center for Medicare and Medicaid Innovation

CMS: Centers for Medicare and Medicaid Services

CNA: Certified nursing assistant

COPD: Chronic obstructive pulmonary disease

CPAP: Continuous positive airway pressure

CPR: Cardiopulmonary resuscitation

DNP: Doctor of Nursing Practice

ELNEC: End-of-Life Nursing Education Consortium

EWA: Eldercare Workforce Alliance

GIP: General In-Patient

HIPAA: Health Insurance Portability and Accountability Act

HPNA: Hospice and Palliative Nurses Association

HUD: U.S. Department of Housing and Urban Development

ICU: Intensive Care Unit

IOM: Institute of Medicine

Appendix B

JAMA: Journal of the American Medical Association

JCAHO: Joint Commission on the Accreditation of Health-care Organizations

LCME: Liaison Committee for Medical Education

LGBT: Lesbian, gay, bisexual and transgender

LPN: Licensed Practical Nurse

MEDPAC: Medicare Payment Advisory Commission

NHPCO: National Hospice and Palliative Care Organization

OAA: Older Americans Act

OBRA: Omnibus Reconciliation Act of 1987

PACE: Program of All-Inclusive Care for the Elderly

PEG: Percutaneous endoscopic gastrostomy tube (also known as a feeding tube)

PCORI: Patient-Centered Outcomes Research Institute

PEAC: Promixis Environment Automation Controller (software that controls the user's environment from wheelchair)

POLST: Physician Orders for Life Sustaining Treatment

SAGE: Services and Advocacy for Gay, Lesbian, Bisexual, and Transgender Elders

VNSNY: Visiting Nurse Service of New York

Acknowledgments

People ask whether I find it depressing to write about issues relating to the end of life. The subject is as serious as, well, a heart attack. My short answer is, no I don't. The biggest reason I don't get depressed is that the people in this realm are simply amazing. Big-hearted, super-smart, passionate about their work, insightful with great energy and even greater sense of humor, they inspire and motivate me. I've been privileged to be in their company.

Holden Caulfield in J.D. Salinger's *Catcher in the Rye* imagined thousands of little kids playing games in a big field of rye while he stands on the edge of "some crazy cliff," as he calls it. All he wants is to catch everybody before they start going over the cliff.

In my research, I imagined these remarkable professionals as grown-up Holden Caulfields dedicated to catching the hordes of elders rolling, shuffling, limping, or otherwise headed toward "that crazy cliff." Their mission is to save them from suffering any more than they already have.

I value the counsel of the many palliative care and hospice physicians, nurses, social workers, advocates for elder care and nursing home transformation who shared their expertise with me. I appreciate their willingness to share their insights, experiences, and hopes about end-of-life care. I am grateful for their encouragement.

Teams of palliative care physicians and nurse practitioners offered me a vision of what the best health care can look like. They are professionals who respect and complement one another, and they are focused on the same goals. As is said about married couples, they often know each other so well and are so comfortable in each other's presence that they finish each other's sentences.

I do owe special thanks to a number of what I've come to think of as All-Stars of palliative and hospice care: F. Amos Bailey, John Balint, Ira Byock, David Casarett, Randall Krakauer, Betty Ferrell, Maribeth Gallagher, Joanne Lynn, Pam Malloy, Joseph Rotella, James Salwitz, Christian Sinclair, Joan Teno, Bill Thomas, Bruce Vladeck, Ann Wyatt. I have unending admiration for Diane E. Meier, the indefatigable and laser-focused head of the Center to Advance Palliative Care.

I am grateful to several editors of medical humanities publications for publishing excerpts adapted from this book: Diane Guernsey and Paul Gross of Pulse—Voices from the Heart of Medicine; Kevin Pho of KevinMD.com; and Randi Belisomo of Life Matters Media. As the late actor Ruth Gordon said, in accepting an Oscar in 1969 at age 72, "I can't tell you how encouraging a thing like this is."

The book would not have become a reality had I not become a hospice volunteer. I am thankful for the patients and families who accepted me in their lives, however briefly. I hope I've brought you a measure of comfort. Thank you to the hospice nurses, social workers, bereavement counselors and chaplains at Holy Name Medical Center for showing that this work can be done with compassion and grace. Long-standing thanks to Sandy Aguece, team manager at Good Shepherd Hospice on Long Island, for coordinating excellent care for my mother, helping to keep me sane during my mother's illness, and introducing me to the real-life benefits of hospice.

I'm grateful to several friends who have read drafts and offered encouragement along with critiques, questions, suggestions, and an eagle-eye for proofreading: Ron, Polly, and Wilma.

Thanks to my husband Ed for his unwavering support and confidence in my ability to do this work, even when he wasn't crazy about the subject matter, and even when I took his editing suggestions with less than good cheer.

My eternal love and thanks go to my son, Matt, my toughest and best critic.

We live in a brave new world of independent publishing, and I am thankful for Bonnie Britt, who not only served as editor, but who also guided me through sometimes daunting aspects of publishing.

About the Cover

I loved the painting "Embrace" from the moment I first saw it featured in the April 4, 2014 edition of the online publication Pulse—Voices from the Heart of Medicine. To me, it is full of life, color and the warmth of human attachment. As such, "Embrace" represents the kindness, compas-

About the Cover

sion and team effort that are the hallmarks of excellent late-life care.

The story behind the painting is striking. It is the art work of Jessica Liu, an Internal Medicine resident physician at Santa Clara Valley Medical Center in San Jose, California. Liu graduated from the University of California, Davis School of Medicine where she served as co-director of the Willow Student-Run Free Clinic.

Liu explained that the clinic holds a weekly Wellness Night at Sacramento's local Salvation Army where temporary shelter residents gather to draw, paint, and meditate. The activity eases some stresses of homelessness. Liu painted alongside the residents, marveling at the way the activity led to open dialogue among strangers. It helped build a sense of community in this vulnerable population. She was moved by people's stories, journeys, struggles and—not least—their talent.

Residents and student doctors alike come and go— both are transient populations—Liu noted, but this experience gave her a lasting appreciation for a holistic approach toward healing.

The painting was subsequently sold as part of a fundraiser for the Clinic. I am grateful to Liu as well as to Angela Rodgers, who now owns the painting, for permitting me to use it for the book cover.

About the Author

Ellen Rand has been a journalist for more than 40 years, including five years as a housing columnist for *The New York Times*. Her essays have appeared in several medical humanities publications, including *Pulse—Voices from the Heart of Medicine; KevinMD;* and *Life Matters Media.* She is a hospice volunteer with Holy Name Medical Center in Teaneck, New Jersey. An avid theater and film fan, she co-founded, and was, for five years, the executive director of a film festival in her community. The theme is "Activism: Making Change." The festival draws an audience of thousands every November.